D1267604

Egypt's Other Wars

Contemporary Issues in the Middle East

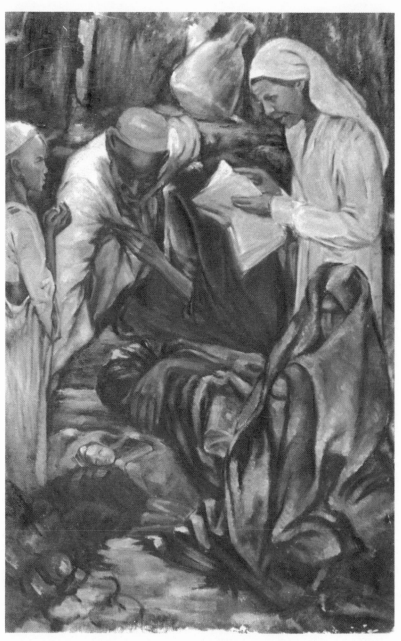

Volunteer interviews the sick in Luxor, 1944. Painting by Amina Sidqi.

Egypt's Other Wars

Epidemics and the Politics of Public Health

Nancy Elizabeth Gallagher

RA
650.8
.E3
G35
1990

Syracuse University Press

Indiana University
Library
Northwest

Copyright © 1990 by Syracuse University Press, Syracuse, New York 13244-5160

All Rights Reserved

First Edition 1990

90   91   92   93   94   95   96   97   98   99   6   5   4   3   2   1

The paper used in this publication meets the minimum requirements of
American National Standard for Information Sciences—Permanence of Paper
for Printed Library Materials, ANSI Z39.48-1984. ∞™

Library of Congress Cataloging-in-Publication Data

Gallagher, Nancy Elizabeth, 1942–
   Egypt's other wars : epidemics and the politics of public health /
Nancy Elizabeth Gallager. —1st ed.
     p. cm.—(Contemporary issues in the Middle East)
   Includes bibliographical references
   ISBN 0-8156-2507-3 (alk. paper)
   1. Epidemiology—Egypt—History.   2. Medical policy—Egypt—
History.   3. Public health—Egypt—History.   I. Title.
II. Series
RA650.8.E3G35   1990
614.4′962—dc   90-31889
                                                 CIP

Manufactured in the United States of America

Contents

Illustrations

Figures

Map

Acknowledgments

The help of many colleagues made writing this book a pleasure. Galal Amin, Raymond Baker, Ali al-Din Hilal Dessouki, Albert Hourani, James Jankowski, Ibrahim Karawan, Kenneth Manning, Afaf Lutfi al-Sayyid Marsot, and Earl L. Sullivan read all or part of the text at different stages and offered useful insights and suggestions. Ralph Jaeckel's scholarly counsel was especially helpful from beginning to end. I would like to thank these and other colleagues who helped directly or indirectly with the manuscript. Any shortcomings are, of course, my own.

While researching the topic I was able to locate many people who had lived through the events under consideration. Many participated in them. I would especially like to thank the following persons: Salah Atiyya, Izdihar Abul Ala Abaza, Layla Barakat, Layla Doss, Muhyi al-Din Farid, Gertrude and Mirit Butrus Ghali, Harry Hoogstraal, Wadud Fayzi Musa, Abd al-Azim Ramadan, Adil Sabit, Fatima Shahin Sabit, and Abd al-Aziz Salah. All shared with me their memories, knowledge, and sometimes their private papers, photographs, and newspaper clippings of the 1940s. It is a privilege to acknowledge their kindness and generosity.

I would like to thank cordially Dunning Wilson and the other librarians and archivists in Egypt, Britain, and the United States who skillfully located numerous primary and secondary materials. They are the unsung heroes of academic research.

Cynthia Maude-Gembler of Syracuse University Press proved an excellent editor. Terresa Ruggieri Joseph and Kathryn Koldehoff carefully copy edited the manuscript.

The cover is a painting by Amina Sidqi done at Luxor in 1944. It depicts a volunteer from the Mabarra Muhammad Ali making a survey of the needs of impoverished malaria victims. I would like to thank

Izdihar Abul Ala Abaza and the Zulficar family of Zamalek for the photographic reproduction.

I am grateful to the American Research Center in Egypt, the Social Science Research Council, the Rockefeller Foundation Archive Center, and the Academic Senate of the University of California, Santa Barbara, for funding this study. I would like to dedicate this book to my husband, Tony, and to our daughter, Lisa Marisol.

Abbreviations and Locations of Manuscript Sources

FO — Foreign Office, Public Record Office, London.

Ghali diary — Diary of Gertrude Butrus Ghali, 1944, privately held by Gertrude Butrus Ghali, Cairo.

Kerr diary — Diary of J. Austin Kerr, 1944–46. R.G. 1.1. Series 485 I. Box 3. Folder 19, Rockefeller Foundation Archives. Rockefeller Archive Center, Tarrytown, N.Y.

Killearn diary — Diaries of Lord Killearn (Sir Miles Lampson), 1942–46, Private Papers Collection, Middle East Centre, St. Antony's College, Oxford.

NA — National Archives and Records Administration, Washington, D.C.

Pridie papers — Papers of Sir Eric Denholm Pridie, (unpublished memoir written in the 1960s), Oriental Section, University Library, Durham University, Durham.

RFA — Rockefeller Foundation Archives, Rockefeller Archive Center, Tarrytown, N.Y.

Soper diary — Diary of Fred L. Soper, 1942–43 and 1944–46. R.G. 12. Box 58. Rockefeller Foundation Archives. Rockefeller Archive Center, Tarrytown, N.Y.

Nancy Elizabeth Gallagher, Associate Professor of History at the University of California, Santa Barbara, is the author of *Medicine and Power in Tunisia, 1780–1900*. After completing her work for an undergraduate degree in public health at the University of California, Berkeley, she earned a doctorate in Middle East history at the University of California, Los Angeles.

Textual Note

To make the story readable, I have intentionally kept transliteration simple and technical terms to a minimum. In most cases I have used the spelling of *Webster's Third New International Dictionary* (e.g., "fellah" rather than "fallah," "tarboosh" rather than "tarbush"). If an Arabic term is not found there, I have followed a simplified version of the transliteration system recommended by the *International Journal of Middle East Studies,* modifying the spelling to reflect Egyptian pronunciation (e.g., "Ebeid" rather than "'Ubayd," "Abaza" rather than "Abadha," "Gamal" rather than "Jamal"). When possible I have eliminated *'ayns* and *hamzas* (e.g., "Muhammad Ali" rather than "Muhammad 'Ali"). I have omitted titles—pasha, bey, hanim, lord, and sir—in all but a few cases.

In 1946 one Egyptian pound (£E) equaled $4.13. One feddan equals 1.038 acres. One *ukka* equals 1.248 kg.

For those unfamiliar with Egyptian geography, Upper Egypt means the southern part and Lower Egypt means the northern part of the country. The Nile flows from south to north, so traveling downriver means traveling north.

Contemporary Issues in the Middle East

Editorial Advisory Board

Roger Allen, *University of Pennsylvania*
John L. Esposito, *College of the Holy Cross*
Yvonne Y. Haddad, *University of Massachusetts*
Tareq Y. Ismael, *University of Calgary*
Kenneth W. Stein, *Emory University*

This well-established series continues to focus primarily on twentieth-century developments that have current impact and significance throughout the entire region, from North Africa to the borders of Central Asia.

Recent titles in the series include:

Development and Social Change in Rural Egypt. Richard H. Adams, Jr.
The Egyptian Bureaucracy. Monte Palmer, Ali Leila, and El Sayed Yassin
Family in Contemporary Egypt. Andrea B. Rugh
Khul-Khaal: Five Egyptian Women Tell Their Stories. Nayra Atiya
The Rise of Egyptian Communism. Selma Botman

Egypt's Other Wars

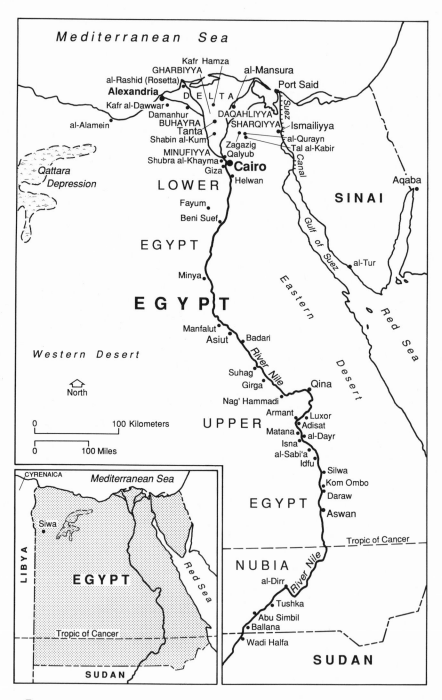

Egypt, 1940s.

I

Introduction

At the beginning of the 1940s public health was a topic of minor importance in Egyptian political life. At the end of the decade it had become an indispensable component of the national political agenda. Public awareness of the crucial importance of public health was aroused by the appearance of severe epidemics of falciparum malaria in 1942–44, relapsing fever in 1946, and cholera in 1947. Other diseases, such as schistosomiasis (bilharzia), ancylostomiasis (hookworm), ophthalmias (trachoma and other eye diseases), tuberculosis, and typhus, also existed before and during the 1940s but did not have the political impact of the malaria, relapsing fever, and cholera epidemics, which occurred during a critical and momentous historical context.[1]

In the 1940s Egypt was in the throes of a nationalistic upheaval. Egyptian nationalists of all political ideologies observed that inhabitants of developed nations rarely suffered from the age-old epidemic diseases because modern science had learned how to prevent and treat them. They attributed the epidemics of the 1940s to Egypt's status as an underdeveloped and colonized nation. The epidemics were therefore not only public health problems but also political problems that called for a political solution. In consequence the epidemics caused a massive mobilization in which King Faruq; majority and minority political parties; elite women volunteers; Islamic, nationalist, and communist groups; British authorities; experts from the Rockefeller Foundation and other international agencies; and, of course, the people in the infected regions all took part. The contenders for power in Egypt sought to win public goodwill not only through their efforts in the public health wars but also through their support for public health reform.

It would have been impossible to trace the events of the epidemics were it not for the lively, expressive, and relatively uncensored Egyptian press of the 1940s. Newspaper editorials, journalists' reports, political cartoons, and diaries revealed political struggles and popular attitudes toward public health reform that are nearly absent from the government's records. Oral interviews with persons who had participated in the events helped answer many questions. The press reports and the oral interviews were checked against the archival and parliamentary records and the secondary accounts. Accuracy can be assumed in none of these sources, but taken together they allow for a judicious reconstruction of Egypt's wars against malaria, relapsing fever, and cholera.

Falciparum malaria (which is sometimes called *malignant malaria*), the first and most severe of the 1940s scourges, is caused by the *Plasmodium falciparum* parasite. The falciparum parasite is carried by the *Anopheles gambiae* mosquito, which likes warm, dark houses and breeds in "shallow, standing, stagnant, sunlit water, sans vegetation" (the five *s*'s memorized by students of malaria). The disease is prevented by mosquito eradication or by using screens, mosquito netting, clothing, and repellents to protect the skin from mosquito bites. Chloroquine phosphate taken orally usually confers protection in regions with infected *A. gambiae* mosquitoes. Patients gradually develop an immunity that is specific to the type of malaria they have experienced. Vaccines are being developed but are still in the experimental stage. Patients with falciparum malaria experience headache and chills followed by a rise in temperature. In severe cases headache, drowsiness, delirium, and confusion can lead to fatalities, especially in nonimmune populations. After about twenty to thirty-six hours the symptoms diminish, and the patient experiences diminished symptoms for three to four days. Untreated falciparum malaria has a high mortality rate, but antimalarial therapy is usually effective. Treatment is with chloroquine except in drug-resistant falciparum malaria, against which quinine and sulfa derivatives are used.[2] Less deadly forms of malaria are caused by three other parasites, *Plasmodium vivax, P. malariae,* and *P. ovale,* which are carried by *Anopheles pharoensis, A. sergenti,* and other anophelene mosquitos. In the 1940s malaria was the most widespread and dangerous disease in the Middle East.[3] All types of malaria are still a threat in large areas of Central and South America, parts of the Caribbean, sub-Saharan Africa, Southeast Asia, and parts of the Middle East.[4]

Relapsing fever, the second of the series of epidemics, is caused by several species of *Borelia* spirochetes, which in Egypt are transmitted most commonly by lice.[5] Relapsing fever thus shares a common vector with typhus but is a very different disease. Typhus, which is endemic in Egypt, strikes suddenly and with very severe symptoms; its survivors are nearly immune to further attacks. Relapsing fever, which is not endemic in Egypt, causes chronic symptoms that can recur for many years unless treated. Patients experience high fever, headache, vomiting, muscle and joint pain, skin rash, and delirium about six days after infection. The symptoms last for about three to five days and recur after a few days of apparent recovery. Mortality is generally low (up to 5 percent), but in epidemics of louse-borne fever cardiac failure may occur and mortality is consequently higher. The disease is prevented by de-lousing with DDT or other insecticides and treated with a single oral dose of tetracycline or erythromycin. Today, with basic hospital care, fatalities are very rare.[6]

Cholera, the third and most famous of the three epidemics, is caused by a vibrio, *Vibrio cholerae,* which is spread by the ingestion of water or food contaminated with the excrement of infected persons. The microbe cannot live outside the human host for more than a few hours, so its presence indicates a symptomatic or an asymptomatic cholera carrier in the vicinity. Patients initially experience diarrhea and vomiting, which often is misdiagnosed as food poisoning. In severe cases water and electrolyte depletion cause intense thirst, muscle cramps, sunken eyes, and wrinkled skin, which becomes black-and-blue from ruptured capillaries. The fatality rate can exceed 50 percent in untreated cases but is less than 1 percent with prompt treatment.

Anticholera vaccines have been sought since Robert Koch's discovery of the *Vibrio cholerae* microbe during Egypt's 1883 epidemic, but the results have generally been disappointing.[7] In 1930, Leonard Rogers, the British cholera expert, reported positive results with the vaccine during a cholera outbreak in India; however, many medical researchers found his results unconvincing because his experiments had not been properly controlled.[8] In 1970 researchers in the Philippines and Bangladesh concluded that the cholera vaccination did not give sufficient protection and that public-health officials should concentrate on upgrading sanitation and therapy centers.[9] Experts today agree that avoidance of contaminated food and water remains the best means of prevention. Cholera is effectively treated with fluid and electrolyte therapy.

Egypt's responses to the epidemics of malaria, relapsing fever, and cholera were shaped by public health policies and political attitudes that had evolved in the nineteenth and early twentieth centuries.[10] In the early nineteenth century, Muhammad Ali (r. 1805–48), an Ottoman military officer, established himself as an Ottoman viceroy following Napoleon's short-lived invasion. He then proceeded to develop Egypt's economy and military forces and recruited a French physician, Antoine Barthèlme Clot (Clot Bey), to design his military and civilian public health services. In the late 1830s the British government, seeking to dominate the eastern Mediterranean, put an end to Muhammad Ali's economic and military expansion. Clot Bey's public health projects, however, continued in attenuated form for many years. In 1882 the British occupied and proceeded to rule Egypt indirectly through Muhammad Ali's descendants and carefully chosen elites. The British authorities' first concern was to reorganize Egypt's finances to collect debts owed to European shareholders. To increase public revenues, British authorities concentrated on agricultural development. British engineers proceeded to expand land under irrigation by harnessing the waters of the Nile. In 1902 they completed a dam at Aswan. The engineers subsequently raised the dam and expanded and reinforced a series of barrages to control better the water flow. Nearly all of Lower Egypt was converted from basin to perennial irrigation so that two or three crops could be grown per year. These agricultural innovations, however, had far-reaching implications for public health conditions in Egypt. When perennial irrigation was expanded in 1902 and 1910, for example, bilharzia, hookworm, and other waterborne diseases spread into formerly uninfected areas of Lower and Middle Egypt. The Egyptian government raised the Aswan dam again in 1933–34. In the late 1930s, when Upper Egypt was being converted from basin to perennial irrigation, the waterborne diseases began to infect the population of Upper Egypt.

Lord Cromer (Evelyn Baring), proconsul and de facto ruler of Egypt from 1882 until 1907, was well aware of the need for medical and public health reform, particularly among the fellahin (peasants), who made up about 70 percent of the population. Most fellahin owned less than ten feddans of land; others rented from large landowners or hired themselves out as migrant workers. In 1883 Clifford Lloyd created the Department of Public Health, a branch of the Ministry of the Interior. Cromer's 1885 report included a study by the newly appointed British surgeon major, who had found that there was only one trained Egyptian doctor for every thirty-two thousand Egyptians and that villagers were relying for medical care on the local barber or midwife who were poorly educated at best. The most common remedies, the surgeon major lamented, were bloodletting, magical charms, and anointment with oil.[11]

Traditional (also called *indigenous* or *empirical*) medicine was considerably more complex than the surgeon major had suggested.[12] Tens of thousands of traditional practitioners provided most of the health care in Egypt. Midwives (*dayas*), health barbers (*halaq al-sihha*s), and certain religious personages (*shaykh*s and *shaykha*s) provided a variety of medical services. Very often charms or amulets were used to ward off disease.[13] As elsewhere in the Middle East, many believed disease and other misfortune could be caused by a glance from a person or even an animal possessing an "evil eye." To protect themselves against the evil eye or other evil spirits people often wore blue beads, the Hand of Fatima or other charms, and amulets containing Quranic inscriptions.[14] *Zar* ceremonies were sometimes held to exorcise harmful spirits from sick persons.

For malaria, health barbers made scratches with cautery needles on the temples, cheeks, or shoulders of their patients to treat the disease.[15] Cautery, bloodletting, and infusions of teas made from powdered sycamore, fenugreek, myrtle, and other leaves were used against the symptoms of fever that were caused by many diseases, including malaria, relapsing fever, and cholera.[16]

During the latter decades of the nineteenth century, many Egyptians, both educated and uneducated, had become aware that modern medicine (also called allopathic, Western, or cosmopolitan medicine) had advanced considerably and, with the discovery of vaccines and microbes, could prevent and treat certain diseases. Beliefs were often combined; people believed that, while microbes caused diseases, supernatural forces selected the individuals the microbes infected. And, while modern medicine could treat certain diseases effectively, so could traditional medicine. As a result, cautery, vaccines, and antibiotics were often used simultaneously. Many believed that traditional remedies were especially effective for joint problems and other chronic complaints, while modern medicine was more effective in treating epidemic diseases and emergency injuries.

These widespread popular beliefs were not reflected in official public health policies. British and Egyptian public health officials alike viewed traditional medical procedures as anachronisms that would disappear in time and rarely considered them in their medical and public health reform plans.[17] At most, sporadic efforts were occasionally made to teach modern medical or nursing techniques to the midwives, health barbers, and other traditional practitioners.[18]

In the 1885 report Cromer said that it was impossible to expect rapid progress in sanitary reform because of a lack of funds. He therefore decided to provide efficient British supervision and gradual education of a "native staff."[19] This policy was to be followed for many years.

In 1892 Secretary of State for the Colonies Alfred Milner wrote that the Department of Public Health was one of the least satisfactory in the government service because, after initial difficulties, "English interest in the matter died away."[20] The department was underfunded and poorly staffed. He complained, "the towns and villages are filthy. The Canals, which are the only sources of water-supply to the bulk of the population, are subject to every kind of pollution. In the neighborhood of many populous places, there are 'birkas,' or stagnant ponds, which exhale miasma even when they are not—as they very often are—used for drinking. In the principal cities there is a certain amount of sweeping and carrying away of refuse, but there is absolutely no drainage. . . . The scope for improvement in sanitary matters at the present time is large enough to give employment for many years to the most ambitious and energetic reformer."[21] Such a reformer did not materialize.

Severe epidemic diseases, however, encouraged the British authorities to strengthen the existing quarantine administration. In 1883, just one year after the British occupation, 58,511 deaths were reported from cholera.[22] French opponents of the British occupation accused the British of having heedlessly imported cholera from India.[23] This accusation was to be repeated in 1947 by Egyptian nationalists. In 1896 and 1902 cholera again struck with devastating results.[24] Pilgrims returning from Mecca had apparently brought the disease into Egypt in each of the epidemics.[25] A series of plague outbreaks occurred from 1898 to 1905. In response British officials reorganized and carefully monitored the quarantine station at al-Tur, a border village in the Sinai. The al-Tur station had been established in 1855 and was used for the first time in 1862.[26] After it was upgraded following the 1902 epidemic, Egypt was free of cholera for many years. Plague outbreaks also diminished in severity.

Although progress was being made in alleviating Egypt's burden of disease, in his 1903 report Cromer acknowledged that, from 1882 to 1903, the British authorities had allocated less than 1 percent of the total state expenditures for sanitation and education.[27] Funds expended by the British authorities came entirely from local taxes and other resources, not from the British government.[28] He lamented the dismal public health and medical conditions that the British found in 1882, but he believed that a few British doctors would be able to "spread the light of Western science throughout the country," even though the school of medicine, founded by Muhammad Ali, had become a "hotbed of ultra-Mohammedan and anti-European feeling."[29] The British doctors were duly employed, but student enrollment in the medical school was severely restricted.

In his 1906 report Cromer quoted from a statement made by the British director of the Qasr al-Ayni medical school, who had cautioned that the number of Egyptians admitted to the school should be carefully controlled. In his opinion, "it is hardly possible to set loose on the country a more dangerous element than the needy medical man."[30] He apparently feared the political and nationalistic activities of Egyptians who were not only unemployed but also well educated. From 1886 to 1890, 112 students graduated from medical school. In the 1890s, as the British took control, the number dropped to ninety-nine from 1891 to 1895 and to only thirty-four from 1896 to 1900.[31] The standards of the school were, however, rapidly brought into line with modern schools in Europe.[32] After 1929, when the school returned to Egyptian administration, the number of graduates was slowly increased. Despite the

increase in graduates the number of trained physicians remained inadequate for Egypt's growing population.[33] *Hakimas* (visiting nurses)
had been trained and licensed since the nineteenth century, but their
numbers were also inadequate.[34]

At the turn of the century adequate medical facilities existed only in
European neighborhoods in Cairo and Alexandria, where, after the
cholera epidemics, British authorities improved the potable water, sew-
age, and sanitation services.[35] The Department of Public Health funded
hospitals that had been established by Muhammad Ali and his grandson
Ismail (r. 1863–79) and introduced numerous improvements. Most of
the better hospitals were, however, privately owned, and each of the
major European communities raised funds and built its own. There
were, for example, Greek, Jewish, Italian, and Anglo-American hospitals. In addition a few Christian missionary societies established hospitals that served the local Egyptian population. American Presbyteri-
ans operated hospitals at Tanta and Aswan and trained Egyptian
women as nurses. After the turn of the century the Department of
Public Health occasionally sent traveling tent hospitals to rural areas
and carried out programs for smallpox vaccination and campaigns
against the eye diseases that afflicted so many Egyptians.[36]

Two Egyptian-run, private, volunteer organizations specialized in
medical care: the Mabarra Muhammad Ali (the Muhammad Ali Benevolent Society) and the Red Crescent Association (Hilal al-Ahmar), the
name taken by International Red Cross organizations in Muslim countries. (Because most of the English-language sources rather contradic-
torily use the name *Mabarra Muhammad Ali* rather than *Muhammad
Ali Benevolent Society* and *Red Crescent* rather than *Hilal al-Ahmar* this
practice will be followed here.) The Mabarra Muhammad Ali was
founded in 1909 by Princess Ayn al-Hayat Ahmad, a member of the
royal family noted for her philanthropic work. She founded a small
dispensary on Muhammad Ali street in one of the poor quarters of the
city. Women of the royal family donated funds from their private incomes to initiate the project. In addition members held concerts and
other functions to raise funds to support medical relief. Over the years
the Mabarra Muhammad Ali established a network of hospitals and
outpatient clinics.[37]

The Egyptian Red Crescent Association was founded in 1912. Its purpose was to extend medical services and aid in times of peace and war and to carry out humanitarian services. Egypt's royal family sponsored and patronized the Red Crescent. Ahmad Fuad (r. 1917–36), youngest son of Ismail and great-grandson of Muhammad Ali, was president of the Red Crescent in the 1910s. Like the Mabarra Muhammad Ali, the Red Crescent established and operated hospitals and clinics in Cairo and Alexandria. The Women's Committee of the Red Crescent Association was founded in 1940 by Nahid Sirri, who had begun her activities by organizing aid for the victims of Turkey's severe earthquake of 1939. Sirri was the aunt of Queen Farida, Faruq's wife, daughter of a former prime minister, Muhammad Sa'id, and wife of Husayn Sirri, a technocratic, pro-British political leader who was prime minister from November 1940 to February 1942. The committee's purpose was to establish a blood bank, to train people in first aid, to make available drugs and equipment for operations, to cooperate with government ministries and departments, and to propagandize the work of the Red Crescent Association. The women's committee raised private funds and also received government grants.[38]

At least one American public health organization was also active in Egypt before World War I. The Rockefeller Foundation, a private American philanthropic organization incorporated in 1910, just before the U.S. Supreme Court broke up the Standard Oil Company of New Jersey, also gave medical assistance to Egypt. The foundation's founders believed that modern medicine was the best means of increasing human happiness and ameliorating human suffering.[39] On the basis of statistics compiled in the United States at the turn of the century, they concluded that public health programs and preventive medicine could reduce sickness by half throughout the world.[40] Scientific medicine could benefit humanity just as science and technology had benefited industry; at the same time, it could promote American interests abroad by winning local appreciation for American assistance and by opening import and export trade.[41] The Rockefeller Foundation's medical experts were impressed by recent discoveries that certain diseases were transmitted by such vectors as snails and mosquitoes. In 1897, for example, Ronald Ross, a British medical researcher, had discovered the role of mosquitoes in malaria transmission.[42] Vector eradication therefore might prove to be an effective means of disease control, and the health of a large portion of the world's population would be vastly improved.[43] Thus, diseases that had been the evils of humanity since the dawn of time could be controlled by the new technical or scientific methods.[44] Malaria was of particular interest to the Rockefeller Foundation because staff members believed it had caused more sickness and death than all other diseases combined.[45] The new foundation formed the International Health Board (later renamed the International Health Division), which carried out disease eradication and other public health projects throughout the world. The International Health Division supported medical research, established training programs for local public health personnel, and gave demonstrations of modern public health and sanitation methods.

In 1913 the foundation made a survey of Lower Egypt and Upper Egypt and found that about 60 percent of the population was infected with hookworm, bilharzia, nonfalciparum malaria, and other parasitic diseases.[46] While Egypt was one of the first countries in which the foundation operated, its projects there were limited to small-scale surveys and pilot studies because its main efforts were concentrated in China, Latin America, and other areas that were then considered to be more important to the United States.

When World War I began, Britain made Egypt a British protectorate, severing its nominal ties with the Ottoman Empire. With British support, Ahmad Fuad, the former president of the Red Crescent, became sultan of Egypt in 1917. During the war the British army requisitioned camels and mules for transport and diverted substantial quantities of wheat, barley, and beans away from the Egyptian food supply to feed its troops. As a result, large numbers of Egyptians became malnourished, and severe epidemics of typhus, typhoid fever, and plague broke out. The deteriorating public health conditions contributed to the growth of nationalistic, anti-British sentiment during the war.

In 1920 a British colonial official, in a memo about ancylostomiasis and bilharzia control, expressed the hope that the rise in political consciousness that Egypt was experiencing might be followed by a corresponding increase in municipal and social responsibility.[47] Egyptian nationalists in turn accused the British authorities of having taken far too little responsibility for the public health and welfare of Egypt.

In 1922 the British government, forced to recognize the strength of

Egyptian nationalism, granted Egypt formal but limited independence. Under the new constitution promulgated in 1923, Ahmad Fuad became king. Sa'd Zaghlul (ca. 1860–1927), leader of Egypt's nationalism movement and head of the Wafd, the recently formed majority political party, was elected prime minister, and Egypt assumed responsibility for its internal affairs, including public health and medicine. Neither the Wafdist nor the non-Wafdist governments of the 1920s and 1930s made more than limited efforts toward social and public health reform, concentrating instead on the three-way power struggle among the palace, the Wafd, and the British that was made inevitable by the weak and divided political system. The Great Depression, however, severely aggravated existing social and economic disparities in Egypt, and in response the Wafd party added an internal social reform program to its nationalistic objectives during its 1935 party congress.[48] The new program called for the creation of village health and educational facilities for the fellahin and for equalized taxation. At that time the poor majority paid a disproportionate share of taxes, while the elite class often paid little or none. In 1936 a Wafd government under Mustafa Nahhas, successor to Sa'd Zaghlul, upgraded the Department of Public Health to the Ministry of Health. The new ministry had eighteen departments, all centralized in Cairo. The Epidemics Section functioned within the Department of Prevention while the Department of Quarantines remained separate.[49] In late 1939 a non-Wafdist government under Ahmad Mahir formed the Ministry of Supplies and the Ministry of Social Affairs.[50] The Ministry of Social Affairs planned to establish rural social centers throughout Egypt.[51] Each center was to contain facilities for health and social welfare, for agricultural extension services, and for local crafts and industries. The ministry took over several soup kitchens run by private social organizations and established additional ones, which encouraged local notables to contribute to them.[52] These projects were, however, limited and afforded only short-term relief for the rural and urban poor. The government also established a Rural Health Section within the Ministry of Health to supervise rural health services. But as Ahmed Zaher Zaghloul of Egypt's High Institute for Public Health succinctly put it in 1963, "few programs were executed and their development was hampered by political and financial reasons."[53]

At the end of the 1930s Egypt was gripped by a severe economic crisis. Small landowners fell into debt and were forced to pay interest rates of 20 to 40 percent. When they could not pay the loans, large landowners bought up their land at advantageous prices, and the former owners joined the underemployed class of landless farm workers or migrated to the cities in search of work. In the cities wages were reduced. Often the cost of living was higher than a full-time urban wage. Yet the large landowners resisted attempts to enact laws or government programs that would have alleviated the misery of the fellahin. Only a few landlords had voluntarily undertaken to provide the fellahin with potable water, satisfactory houses, or health facilities.

A Rockefeller Foundation survey made in 1939 found that malaria was much more prevalent in Lower Egypt than had been thought. This was a relatively mild form of malaria carried principally by the *A. pharoensis* mosquito rather than the more severe falciparum malaria carried by the *A. gambiae* mosquito found in sub-Saharan Africa and elsewhere.[54] Shortly after World War I the Rockefeller Foundation had begun to specialize in mosquito eradication projects and further developed its techniques in numerous projects in many regions of the world in the 1920s and 1930s. The foundation was considering a malaria eradication project in Lower Egypt when war again broke out in Europe and diverted attention to the war effort.[55]

Egypt was immediately caught up in World War II. Britain was able to expand its military presence there under the terms of a treaty signed in 1936, when the threat of world war in general and the Italian expansion in Africa in particular had forced the two nations to work out their differences. Under the terms of the 1936 Treaty, Britain could in wartime expand its military bases and have unrestricted use of Egyptian land, water, and airspace but could in peacetime station no more than ten thousand troops there and these only in the Canal Zone.[56] By the end of 1939 Cairo was full of Allied troops defending the Suez Canal and the eastern Mediterranean against the Axis powers, which were mobilizing to attack from Cyrenaica. About three hundred thousand British army troops—mostly from Britain and Australia but also from South Africa, New Zealand, and other parts of the empire—were stationed in Egypt.[57] The British barracks in Cairo was located in the center of town on the site where the Nile Hilton now stands. Tal al-Kabir, located in the Canal Zone, was the largest British base in the Middle East.[58]

Most Egyptians considered the war a European affair and hoped to avoid being drawn into it. Some hoped for a German victory, which might rid them at last of the British occupation. All feared a repetition of the famines and epidemics that had occurred during World War I. A few Egyptian medical experts hoped the war would bring an opportunity for the introduction of much-needed public health reform.

In 1940 Abd al-Wahid al-Wakil, an Oxford-trained professor of hygiene in the faculty of medicine of Fuad al-Awal University and a former inspector of public health in Cairo, called for the formation of *wahdat mujamma'at* (social service units) which could expand health and social services to the fellahin.[59] Wakil's comments were unusually important because of his political connections. His niece, Zaynab al-Wakil, had recently married Mustafa Nahhas, and Wakil and the rest of his family had become active Wafdists. The following year at a major address at the American University in Cairo, Wakil told his audience that 75 percent of the Egyptian people were afflicted with bilharzia, 50 percent with ancylostomiasis, 50 percent with other parasitic diseases, 90 percent with trachoma, 15 percent with malaria, 7 percent with pellagra, and all with numerous childhood diseases. Life expectancy was thirty-one years for men and thirty-six years for women. He compared these rates with those in Britain, where life expectancy was fifty-five for men and fifty-nine for women. The mortality rate in Egypt had risen from 25.3 per thousand at the beginning of century to 26.5 per thousand in 1941 despite 118 years of sanitary organization. In Britain during the same period, it had fallen from 16 per thousand to 12 per thousand. The situation was, he said, growing worse instead of better: overall mortality in the past fifteen years had increased by 5 percent, child mortality by 15 percent. Because poverty was the cause of the poor health conditions, he advocated more equitable distribution of land and prohibition of extensive landholdings. Only the government had the power to undertake the necessary reforms in the economic system. In the meantime, Egypt needed more hospitals and public health facilities.[60] He clearly intended that a future Wafdist government would implement his ideas for public health reform.

It was not, however, an auspicious time for the reform of Egypt's public health services. The future was not at all clear. In February 1942 Rommel's Afrika Korps had advanced to within seventy miles of Alexandria and was planning to occupy the city before pressing on to Suez. Egyptian foreboding was correct: the war effort had aggravated the existing economic problems in Egypt and elsewhere in the Middle East. The British government took steps to avoid a repetition of the crises of World War I. When Germany occupied France, took positions in North Africa, and sent reinforcements to the Italians in Libya, the Mediterranean Sea was closed to commercial shipping; Egypt and most of the Middle East were suddenly cut off from their normal supply routes. The British military purchased large quantities of Egyptian cereals and cotton to supply the hundreds of thousands of Allied troops based in Egypt. In 1941–42 there were shortages of all basic foodstuffs. People began hoarding wheat and fuel, scarcity drove prices up, and the poor were unable to afford adequate food and clothing. A flourishing black market encouraged profiteering and enabled only the wealthy to buy provisions. Rumors of hoarding and of bakers who mixed sawdust and flour to make bread were whispered from person to person. The public blamed both the British military for buying up Egypt's supplies and the Egyptian government for allowing the supplies to be sold. The government put through a law guaranteeing the fellahin food for themselves and fodder for their animals for three months, but relief was only temporary.[61] In 1941 the British government established the Middle East Supply Centre in Cairo to procure military and civilian supplies for the region, but it was not able to offset entirely the shortages caused by the war. In early 1942 the Middle East Supply Centre received word that the wheat and barley in Egyptian storehouses would not last past spring. British authorities were forced to return part of the purchased grain.[62] The fellahin were, however, forced to pay increased prices for the additional supplies. Consequently, while those who worked for the British forces earned increased salaries and war profiteering made a few entrepreneurs wealthy, rural conditions worsened, especially in Upper Egypt.

Meanwhile, King Faruq, who had succeeded his father Fuad in 1936, hoped the war would enable him to get rid of British tutelage. Faruq was then a handsome young man of twenty-two and enormously popular with his subjects. He resented British dominance; in particular he resented the condescending manner of the British ambassador, Miles Lampson (hereafter, Lord Killearn, which he was called after he was made a peer in January 1943).[63] Faruq and several government officials made indirect contacts with Britain's Italian and German opponents in anticipation of a British defeat.

Lord Killearn was one of the last great imperialists and was indeed authoritarian and condescending in style, especially to Faruq, whom he considered a nuisance.[64] Killearn was aware that Faruq, officials in the Egyptian government, and military officers were trying to subvert the British war effort. Killearn considered their attitudes and activities disloyal, and he sought to find a way to depose Faruq and to install a pro-British government. Having obtained approval from Anthony Eden, then foreign secretary, he made his move.[65] On 4 February 1942 British tanks surrounded Abdin Palace. Killearn met with Faruq and presented him with an ultimatum: appoint a government headed by Mustafa Nahhas or abdicate. After consultation with his counselors and former prime ministers, Faruq complied. It was clear that the British still made and unmade governments despite Egypt's official independence from Britain. The credibility of the Wafd party as the leading nationalist party had been damaged because, though it had long based its credentials on its inflexible opposition to British dominance, it had accepted British support in coming to power. For its part, the Wafd believed that it had been out of power too long, owing to palace interference, and that, being the majority party, it had the right and obligation to rule. Faruq and his palace entourage now sought to turn the tables against the Wafd government.

Among the public anti-British sentiment ran dangerously high. In February 1942, for example, Egyptian medical students marched in demonstrations carrying signs urging Rommel onward. Mrs. Garvice, a British doctor who had been employed by the Egyptian government for many years, mentioned to an embassy official that the majority of the Egyptian intelligentsia and 90 percent of the medical students were not only anxious to see Great Britain defeated but actually wanted the Germans to come to Egypt. The Germans and their scientific methods would quickly stamp out bilharzia and hookworm in contrast with the British, who, the students said, had never attempted to deal with these diseases.[66]

Garvice's comments were written up and circulated among the embassy staff. Embassy First Secretary Michael Wright believed there was much truth in her observations. Before he arrived, he had been under the impression that the British had done much to improve the health of Egyptians. He had tried hard since arriving to find out exactly what the British had done, but he could find no one who knew the details. The British certainly did not use their public health contributions to Egypt as a propaganda weapon. He thought that with the Wafd back in power the time might be right for large-scale British aid. It would result in the infiltration of British medical influence into towns and villages up and down Egypt.[67]

Walter Smart, counselor to the British embassy, regretted that the British had done nothing to fill in the *birka*s (pools of standing water) found in most villages of Egypt and had left bilharzia control to the Rockefeller Foundation. He recommended that the British work toward establishing a medical research institute on the lines of the Rockefeller Foundation. The real cause of the public health problem was, he insisted, the wretched condition of the fellahin, a social problem with which the British could not cope. He concluded that the surest way to make Egyptians healthier would be to destroy the dams the British had built and return to basin irrigation. After half of the population had died of hunger, he said, the rest would be healthier.[68]

Lawrence Grafftey-Smith, head of the publicity section of the embassy and former Orient secretary, believed that the British record in public health was good and favorably recalled in Egypt. He warned in his report that real improvement in public health meant not injections but changes in the living conditions of the fellahin, introduction of basic sanitation facilities, availability of potable water, and instruction in elementary hygiene. He recalled that William Willcocks, the British engineer who had designed the first Aswan Dam, had prophesied that perennial irrigation would ruin the health of Egyptians by raising the subsoil water level, and he remembered that Thomas Russell, British chief of police in Cairo from 1902 to 1946, had drawn a connection between irrigation and drug abuse because drugs imparted a sense of stamina that mitigated the debilitating effects of bilharzia and hookworm.[69]

Grafftey-Smith favored the idea of a research institute and suggested that, although Egyptians were sensitive about "grants from foreign bodies," the matter might be brought up with Mustafa Nahhas, the

Wafdist prime minister the British had just installed in office. He added in a postscript that he must say that Mrs. Garvice was one of the most dangerous talkers in the British community.[70]

While Egyptians seethed with nationalistic resentment, the British embassy worried about Egyptian loyalties, and the British military authorities prepared to defend the Suez Canal, a silent and unseen enemy was invading Upper Egypt and taking up positions in two of its provinces. Egypt would have to fight.

2

Malaria Invades

In April 1942 the Ministry of Health in Cairo received reports from Abu Simbil and Ballana, both small towns in Aswan province, that an unidentified epidemic was decimating their populations. The towns were near the Sudanese border in the center of Nubia.[1] The ministry sent Sadallah Madwar, its medical entomologist, to investigate. He left Cairo 30 April, traveled by ship up the Nile, and arrived in Abu Simbil on 5 May. He found the town deserted. There were no people in the streets. The schools were closed because the children and teachers were all sick. The people were suffering from an irregular, intermittent fever. The ministry had at first suspected yellow fever, so its workers took two hundred thick-drop blood smears and examined them in Abu Simbil. All were positive for falciparum malaria.

Madwar wired Cairo for help. Two other medical workers soon arrived with a shipload of antimalarial drugs. The boat crew had to unload the medicine themselves because the townspeople were too ill to work. Two hundred people had already died in the two towns, and smaller villages in Nubia reported thousands of cases. The health authorities checked school registers and concluded from absentee rates that the epidemic had begun in February or March and had worsened in April. The medical workers began distributing the medicine house-to-house. For two weeks they worked without stop, visiting the sick and passing out the antimalarial drugs. Sometimes they had to travel thirty kilometers by donkey to reach the sick in remote areas.[2]

In May Madwar went to Wadi Halfa, a town just over the Sudanese border, to visit a malaria station. There a British entomologist showed him mosquitoes that had been bred from *Anopheles gambiae* larvae collected in May 1941 from river pools along the banks of the Nile a few miles south of the Egyptian border. Soon after, Madwar found *A. gambiae* larvae at Abu Simbil. On 29 June he telegraphed the news to the Ministry of Health: *A. gambiae* had established themselves and had begun breeding in Upper Egypt.[3]

The Ministry of Health was not prepared to deal with an epidemic of falciparum malaria in Upper Egypt. When the Department of Health became the Ministry of Health in 1936, a new Malaria Section had been established in response to an increase in malaria carried by the *A. pharoensis* vector, but this was nonfalciparum malaria, a much less deadly form. In 1942 the Malaria Section had only six doctors, all of whom worked in the Fayum and the Suez Canal Zone where nonfalciparum malaria was endemic. The annual budget of the Malaria Section was only £E 5,000 to 8,000 (the Egyptian pound was then worth about five dollars). With the new threat, the budget was immediately raised to £E 10,000 and at the end of 1942 to £E 50,000.

Khalil Abd al-Khaliq, the director of the Institute of Tropical Medicine in Cairo who had just been appointed undersecretary of health for quarantine administration, sent Muhyi al-din Farid, a malaria expert, to the region to make a survey of the gambiae mosquito foci (fig 1). Abd al-Khaliq's duties were to discover and combat infectious diseases and to safeguard the country against the introduction of epidemic disease, especially plague and cholera, from outside Egypt.[4] Like many of his generation, he very much resented foreign interference in Egypt's internal affairs. In his new position as head of the quarantine administration, Abd al-Khaliq frequently and vociferously linked epidemiological crises to political problems.

In July 1942 Farid found the mosquito in the towns of Aswan, Kom Ombo, Daraw, and Idfu. In August he found it in Luxor and Girga, in September in Asiut, and in November in Manfalut. Mosquitoes carrying malaria parasites were slowly moving downriver toward the Delta, where the river split into thousands of canals, where millions of Egyptians lived, and where hundreds of thousands of Allied troops were mobilized for the war with Rommel's Afrika Korps.

Because falciparum malaria was not normally found in Egypt, the

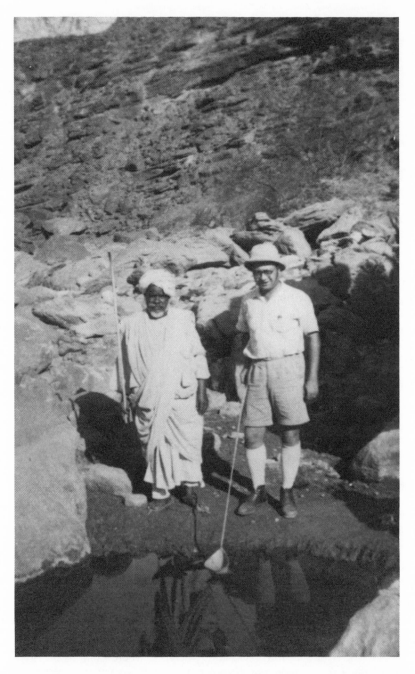

Fig. 1. Muhyi al-Din Farid and a leader of the Bashariya (nomadic inhabitants of Upper Egypt) searching for *Anopheles gambiae* larvae near Aswan. Photograph taken in 1943. Courtesy Muhyi al-Din Farid.

mosquitoes that transmitted the disease must have arrived in Egypt already infected with the deadly parasite. But how were the mosquitoes brought in to Egypt? *A. gambiae* mosquitoes were endemic in Sudan and in West Africa, but not in Egypt. From the start of the outbreak Egyptian authorities had accused the British army of importing the mosquito via military transport. In 1942 when the Mediterranean route was closed to overflight, military planes flew an alternate route to Egypt via Takoradi in West Africa and Sudan.[5] Abd al-Khaliq claimed that the *A. gambiae* mosquito had been carried into Egypt from West Africa by British military aircraft. The Egyptian government threatened to demand war reparations from the British government for damages caused by the outbreak.

Malaria experts accordingly made every effort to learn the source of the epidemic. Khalil Abd al-Khaliq was certain that falciparum malaria had never before occurred in Egypt. Major Theodore, a British military malaria expert who was investigating the outbreak, believed there had been many such outbreaks of falciparum malaria in Upper Egypt.[6] If proven, this would tend to exonerate the British military aircraft of having brought the malaria mosquito to Upper Egypt. Furthermore, if the disease habitually crossed over from Sudan without spreading to Lower Egypt, the danger to Allied troops might be exaggerated.

To ascertain the truth, malaria experts interviewed elderly persons in towns throughout Upper Egypt asking them if they had experienced such severe malaria in the past. They said they had indeed. Many people connected the malaria outbreaks to the expansion of irrigation. People recalled that in 1905 when the Kom Ombo sugar planation opened, malaria had broken out. Further questioning suggested that the outbreak was probably not falciparum malaria transmitted by gambiae but rather the more benign type transmitted by the local anopheles mosquitoes.[7] After the first raising of the dam in 1912, there was an outbreak of falciparum malaria in Wadi al-Arab north of Nubia. After a heavy rainfall in 1919–20 in al-Dirr, a town in central Nubia, water had been standing for several months, and there had been a brief outbreak of malaria. About a thousand people had perished in a very short time. When the flood receded, the epidemic had vanished.[8]

In 1933–34 the Aswan dam was raised again. Pumps were introduced into Nubia to convert formerly basin-irrigated land into perennially irrigated land. Again, there was more standing water to allow for the expansion of sugarcane cultivation. An outbreak of falciparum malaria had stricken the population of Tushka following the expansion of perennial irrigation.[9]

In early 1942, however, the mosquito had established itself for the first time in Upper Egypt and had begun to breed and spread further downriver. The expansion of perennial irrigation in the late 1930s had apparently created the conditions for the mosquito to survive the winter. In some of the villages he had visited during his January 1943 survey, the villagers declared emphatically that they had never before experienced falciparum malaria because it was far more widespread than it had been in the past.

D. J. Lewis, a British malaria expert, considered the possibility that military aircraft had transported the mosquito from West Africa to Sudan and then to Egypt. He noted that most military aircraft flew from Sudan directly to Cairo. If British planes from Khartoum had carried the mosquito into Egypt, the disease should have broken out around Cairo, but it did not. Furthermore, aircraft departing from Sudan took off from an airport several kilometers from the Nile where no gambiae had been found. Aswan, the capital of Upper Egypt, did not have an airport in 1942. The British did have a small landing strip at Tushka, but it was in the desert and was infrequently used.[10]

Muhyi al-Din Farid subsequently made the unexpected finding that gambiae could breed on a water plant (*Potamogeton crispus*) that grew in the Nile in thick matlike formation. Farid's discovery led the experts to conclude that malaria-infected mosquitoes had been brought downriver to Egypt by boat and had then begun breeding and traveling on the water plants.[11] Fred L. Soper, an American Rockefeller Foundation expert, doubted Farid's discovery and made him a five-piaster bet that it was not so. Soper duly paid him the five-piaster note, which had the words "you won" written on the edge.[12]

Aswan was two hundred miles north of Wadi Halfa, where malaria had long been endemic, but the banks of the Nile between Aswan and Wadi Halfa formed a natural barrier between Sudan and Egypt. The banks were steep, rocky, and barren and had no likely breeding places.[13] However, steamers and feluccas frequently plied the route carrying large clay pots loaded with wheat and other cargo, and river transport was greatly increased during the war. The clay pots were stacked and tied to the decks of the boats, with their necks open and facing outward. The gambiae mosquitoes, liking warm, dark places, probably sought refuge in the jars and were comfortably transported into Egypt.[14]

Most Egyptian, British, and American malaria experts came to agree that the gambiae mosquito had probably entered Egypt by ship, had established itself in the shallow pools of standing water around Aswan, and had spread from there.[15] Nevertheless, many nationalistic Egyptians continued to insist that British military aircraft had brought the malaria mosquito into Egypt.

Malaria waned as the weather grew warmer and the Nile receded, but malaria workers warned local *umdas* (village mayors appointed by the central government) that the situation could become serious later in the year, when the annual Nile flood would again create numerous potential breeding sites. The workers gave the *umdas* supplies of antimalarial drugs to distribute in case of further outbreaks and told them to fill in the *birkas* that were located near most villages since they were ideal breeding places for mosquitoes.[16] The *birkas* were formed by natural water seepage and by drainage from nearby villages and were used as water holes for animals, as ponds for ducks, and as wading pools for children. Efforts to drain them were halfhearted at best.

Later that year the Nile rose and receded as it had since the beginning of time. Pools of standing water were everywhere. Borrow pits, dug to raise land for the railroad tracks, collected stagnant water. Water seeped into holes where fellahin had taken mud to make bricks and into footprints and hoofprints left in the soft earth. Summer was too hot for the adult mosquitoes to be active, but in September, October, and November millions of young *A. gambiae* mosquitoes lifted off from the standing pools.

Provincial governors frantically wired Cairo for help. Fellahin in many regions were soon too sick to work, and in October and November about half the land lay fallow. Ministry of Health workers again returned to Upper Egypt and again gave out quantities of antimalarial drugs to *umdas* for distribution. Transportation and medical facilities were limited, and ministry doctors were able to treat only a few of the cases. Because many in the region were also suffering from malnutrition, Ministry of Health officials began to distribute food supplies. By the end of December 1942 when the epidemic had waned, many thousands of persons had perished: some villages were devastated; others were entirely spared.

Despite the severity of the outbreak, news of it had not reached Cairo. Occasionally *al-Ahram,* the most respected newspaper in Egypt, published brief notices that Abd al-Wahid al-Wakil, who had become minister of health in the new Wafdist government, and other officials had left Cairo to tour Upper Egypt.[17] No reason for such trips was mentioned in the announcements, but subsequent events revealed their connection with the epidemic. Was the Wafd government concealing the outbreak?

On 1 December 1942 Wakil gave a speech in Cairo, comparing health conditions in World War I and World War II. He said that, to the credit of his ministry, the current incidence of disease such as typhus and plague, was much less than during World War I.[18] There was an outbreak of malaria in Upper Egypt, he admitted, but it was the result of an exceptionally heavy flood that would have been averted had the Wafd party been able to stay in power and complete irrigation and electrification projects begun in 1936, after the Aswan Dam was raised.[19] He implied that the completed projects would have raised the standard of living in Upper Egypt and would have enabled the population to withstand the effects of the malaria outbreak.

Again on 9 December 1942 the press announced that Wakil had departed on a two-week tour of Nubia to supervise the distribution of maize, oil, and sugar.[20] Again no reason was given, and neither famine nor malaria was mentioned.

The Wafd government, which had recently come to power in the most dubious of circumstances, had apparently decided to minimize and partially censor news of the epidemic to protect itself from criticism. Furthermore, Robin Furness, the British wartime military censor in Egypt, had issued a regulation in 1941 prohibiting publication of information or statistics about any epidemic disease in Egypt without his express approval.[21] The British did not want the Axis forces to know if epidemic diseases threatened Allied troops. Both the British and the Egyptian authorities were happy to have the epidemic kept out of the news.

Suppression of news of epidemic diseases is not uncommon. The opposition can criticize the government for failing to provide for public welfare. Trade and commerce can be hindered. Public fears may contribute to social and political upheaval. Under certain historical conditions epidemics and other natural disasters can cause social upheavals and popular revolts and can lead to the overthrow of governments.[22]

Wakil was preoccupied with a new public-health program. In 1942 the government had promulgated the "Improvement of Village Health Law," which called for the creation of a health unit for every thirty thousand people. The initial plan was for 850 units.

In the summer and fall of 1942, the British authorities were in no position to concern themselves with a malaria outbreak in Upper Egypt because Allied troops based in the Delta were preparing for the final battle for Egypt and Suez, and it was far from clear that the British would be able to stay in Egypt at all. A defeat might have cut access to the Soviet Union and India, allowed Germany and Japan to link up, and led to a German and Italian occupation of northern and northwestern Africa.[23] After the decisive Allied victory at al-Alamein on 22 October 1942, the British military authorities believed at first that the outbreak would remain confined to one or two provinces of Upper Egypt.

In November 1942 American troops entered the war in North Africa and Egypt. Intense American interest in Egypt dates from about 1941, when Roosevelt declared that the Middle East was of vital importance to the United States. To secure the Allied powers' access to its oil reserves, he committed the United States to the defense of the region against German expansion. Also in November 1942, President Roosevelt issued an executive order establishing the U.S.A. Typhus Commission, which was to monitor, study, and prevent the recurrence of the typhus epidemics that had decimated troops during World War I. The commission's headquarters were immediately set up in Abbasiyya, a suburb of Cairo, next to the Egyptian government's Infectious Fever Hospital. The commission's facilities for scientific research in typhus and other infectious diseases soon became the most advanced in the Middle East. The commission's members were from the U.S. Army and Navy Medical Corps, the U.S. Public Health Service, and the Rockefeller Foundation.

In January 1943 Fred L. Soper, the above-mentioned Rockefeller

Foundation expert, came to Egypt with the typhus commission to which he had been seconded. Between 1938 and 1940 Soper and Bruce Wilson, a Canadian malaria expert, had directed a successful *A. gambiae* control program in Brazil. In the early 1930s the mosquito had been air transported from West Africa to Brazil, where it had established itself for the first time. In Brazil, malaria had already stricken one hundred thousand people and had caused fourteen thousand deaths when the control program began, but within months the Rockefeller experts and their Brazilian colleagues administered an effective vector eradication campaign.[24] Soper was convinced that he could administer an equally effective campaign in Egypt.

The Malaria Section of the Ministry of Health invited Soper to one of its meetings, where he described the gambiae eradication project he had directed in Brazil. Soper hoped that the ministry would invite the Rockefeller Foundation to direct a similar project in Egypt, but he decided that no one at the meeting was interested. Khalil Abd al-Khaliq was, he found, especially hostile to his offer.[25] Soper, however, did receive permission from the Ministry of Health to go upriver to make a survey of the malaria region. The ministry asked Muhyi al-Din Farid, who had worked with the Rockefeller Foundation in Egypt in the 1930s, to accompany him. The two researchers reached Girga, the midpoint of the malaria-infected region. Upon their return, Soper submitted a report of his findings to the Ministry of Health, the American legation, and the British embassy.

In the report, Soper said that gambiae was well distributed in Upper Egypt, was still spreading, and posed a genuine threat to Lower Egypt. He recommended that the ministry establish an emergency, temporary gambiae eradication service with adequate funding, led by a director who could hire and fire workers. Such a service should use Paris green for disinfecting standing water and pyrethrum for disinfecting boats, trains, and cars.[26]

The director of the typhus commission, C. S. Stephenson, wrote Soper to say that he believed the Egyptians would "make a mess of this gambiae job."[27] He said that if the malaria mosquito did invade the Nile Delta, it would be one of the "world's unnecessary tragedies."[28] People would have to be evacuated, and it would hinder the war effort. He said he thought there was "a great deal more political than biological science" involved in the Egyptian government's efforts to handle malaria control themselves.[29] Nevertheless, Soper concluded that the Egyptian government authorities had put too much money and effort into the antigambiae program itself and that it would not want the Rockefeller Foundation to take over its management.[30] When Ali Tawfiq Shusha, permanent undersecretary of health, sent a note to him thanking him for his survey of the gambiae-infected region and assuring him that the procedures he had recommended were consistent with those already being applied by the ministry, he concluded that this was a negative response to his recommendation. He was very pessimistic and anticipated another epidemic of malaria later in 1943.[31] After a second survey in April, he made one more attempt to secure an invitation to form a gambiae eradication service, but nothing came of it.[32]

Killearn meanwhile recommended that British army malaria experts be dispatched to assist the Egyptians. He thought such assistance would mitigate the Egyptian government's allegations that British military aircraft had transported the malaria mosquito into Egypt.[33] But before authorizing the assistance, British military authorities wanted to know if there was a genuine danger of malaria spreading to Lower Egypt, where most of their troops were based. If there was no danger, they preferred to give priority to military needs in combat areas.[34] The Middle East Supply Centre in Cairo replied that there was indeed danger to Allied troops and that, if no help was given and malaria spread in 1943, the Egyptian government and people would almost certainly blame the British.[35]

The Middle East Supply Centre acted as a sort of mediator between the British embassy and the British military authorities, because it straddled the civilian and military worlds.[36] This position was important because the embassy and the military had somewhat different interests: the embassy was concerned with the local political scene and with public opinion, while the military was concerned with the war effort.

In early 1943 the Middle East Supply Centre and the British Minister of State formed the Middle East Medical Advisory Committee to provide technical assistance to local health authorities and medical experts to advise in antiepidemic campaigns. Soper played a dominant role in this committee, and his views prevailed in its decision to allocate shipping tonnage for the importation of the supplies of Paris green requested by the Ministry of Health.[37]

Killearn became worried about Soper's presence. Wakil, the minister of health, had "recently confidentially informed the Embassy of an attempt by the American Minister to secure a contract for Dr. Soper, the American Malaria expert, without our being previously informed."[38] This move was irregular because Egypt was a British, not an American, sphere of influence. He explained to Anthony Eden, then foreign secretary, that Wakil was "averse to the employment of Americans in general and of Dr. Soper in particular."[39] British medical authorities, he said, were willing to cooperate with American experts but feared "that such cooperation would be stultified by the uncompromising personality of Dr. Soper."[40] He concluded that despite the British general headquarters having said that climatic conditions made the spread of the mosquito to the Delta unlikely, the political aspect now required the British to take action.[41] When Soper had proposed that the Rockefeller Foundation take over the malaria campaign, Killearn had recommended against it. Killearn's recommendation had considerable weight since the newly established Wafd government was dependent upon British support. Soper had assured Killearn that the Rockefeller Foundation was a private organization with no connections with U.S. military forces, but Killearn did not find this distinction reason to change his mind.

The threat of American involvement in Egyptian public-health issues led the British embassy to reconsider its role in public-health work. Walter Smart, Orient counselor to the British embassy, was asked to prepare a memorandum on health conditions in Egypt for the foreign office.[42] In the memorandum he acknowledged that the health of Egypt was now generally considered worse than it had been before the British entered in 1882.[43] The picture was ominous: if the British were unable to contribute to improving Egypt's health problems, "international enterprise" might interest itself in Egypt. The Rockefeller Foundation had already been carrying out bilharzia research on a small scale for many years and might expand its activities. The entry of falciparum malaria into Upper Egypt illustrated the inadequacy of the Ministry of Health in dealing with such epidemics. Smart believed that a British research institute, where researchers would study means of controlling endemic and epidemic diseases, would introduce British methods into the field of Egyptian health. He concluded, "Nothing could do more for British influence in Egypt, there could be no more powerful form of propaganda, than a successful British effort to improve the health of a malady-stricken country." The institute would also draw Egyptian and British scientists into "close, unpolitical contacts." In closing, he suggested that the decline of British influence in Egypt had been largely attributable to the decline of personal contacts between British and Egyptian officials.[44]

As usual the memorandum was circulated for comments among the embassy personnel before being sent to the foreign office. One commentator said that it was regrettable that the British public conscience had to be prompted by American political ambitions: an Anglo-American contest in public service was distasteful to contemplate. He recommended that the British either let the Americans go ahead with their plans or establish the medical research institute. Another said that, whether the British let the Americans go ahead with their plans or cooperated with them, the Americans would still get all the credit. Therefore if the British were able to deal with Egypt's public health problems, they should simply tell the Americans that the job was already being done.[45] This choice of words indicates a quite remarkable tendency to consider the Egyptian government a simple observer in matters of public health, despite its medical corps, its Ministry of Health, and its other public health facilities.

In a cover letter accompanying the memorandum and comments submitted to Anthony Eden, Killearn warned that future prospects looked gloomy unless the British tackled Egypt's health problems energetically and scientifically. Otherwise, he said, the Americans might step in and do the job.[46] But what seemed of paramount importance in Cairo seemed less so in London. Eden took no action. In the spring of 1943 the war in North Africa had gone in favor of the Allies, but elsewhere it was far from over. It was not the time to consider long-term medical assistance projects in Egypt.[47]

Meanwhile, public health matters seemed to take a turn for the better. On 16 May 1943 the ministry announced that there had been no cases of malaria in Aswan province that season because of the efforts of the malaria-control station. Workers had successfully disinfected wells, drainage canals, and other bodies of standing water.[48] At the beginning of the summer control work in the malaria zone was at a standstill. The ministry had concluded that malaria was under control.

That assessment soon proved premature. Early in the fall of 1943, people throughout Upper Egypt began showing symptoms of malaria. Soon people in towns and villages throughout Qina and Aswan provinces were prostrate from malaria. By mid-October conditions had so deteriorated that gambiae eradication workers left their posts and began frantically to distribute Atabrine. Fields that had been full of fellahin working the land were now vacant. Kom Ombo, a town and region of about forty thousand inhabitants and a center of the modern sugar industry, was severely stricken.[49] The manager of the Kom Ombo sugar plantation estimated that 99 percent of the people were sick and said that he himself had three recurrences of malaria in 1942 and 1943. He told malaria workers that area villages, which usually had six or seven deaths per month, now had sixty or seventy. British and American military authorities supplied the Ministry of Health with enough Atabrine to treat one-half million cases of malaria.[50] Kom Ombo later reported five thousand deaths from malaria.[51]

In the Idfu region of Upper Egypt many communities reported 100 percent of the population ill. The local doctor in al-Sabi'a (al-Sibi'iyya), a small town in the region, had four recurrences. The director of the Amiri (government) hospital in Isna and his family all contracted malaria. Local authorities estimated that 50 percent of the population of Upper Egypt had contracted the disease. The epidemic had begun in September, worsened in October, November, and December, and waned in January. A graph made in Isna suggested that gambiae had been in the region in small numbers in 1942 but had consolidated its hold in 1943, when deaths were much more numerous.[52]

In Matana, where Faruq owned estates, the peak month was October, when nearly the entire population was stricken. The manager of the king's estates said that local authorities had been able to obtain ample quantities of medicines in 1942, when about 1 percent of the population had been ill, but had been unable to do so in 1943, when control and treatment procedures had completely broken down.[53]

In Armant, the local doctor had apparently misdiagnosed malaria as influenza and had suspended all antimalaria therapy for two weeks.

Deaths rose to eighty or ninety persons per day. Sadallah Madwar, the Ministry of Health's medical entomologist, reported having seen coffins being carried away all day. The manager of the Abbud sugar plantation estimated that 80 to 90 percent of the people had contracted malaria.[54] In every affected region, only the poverty-stricken perished. Virtually all of the ministry workers and more affluent inhabitants who contracted malaria recovered. The connection between poverty and disease was apparent to all.

The economic consequences of the malaria epidemic were catastrophic. People who had the disease could not work, and even when they began to recover, their work capacities were much reduced by relapses and long convalescences. With diminished incomes, they were further weakened, and many suffered serious relapses and often contracted other diseases. It took ten men to do the work usually done by five. Employers had to pay migrant workers five times the salary of local workers, and they also contracted malaria. The result was a substantial reduction in wheat and sugar crops in Upper Egypt in 1943 and a substantial increase in malnutrition.[55] In many areas, the wheat crop was not brought in, and about one-third of the sugar crop was lost.[56] The 1944 wheat crop in Upper Egypt was also exceptionally poor since the lack of farm labor had impeded planting.[57] Ministry of Health officials later estimated that the total economic loss was about £E 4 million.[53] Crop production in Lower Egypt for 1943 and 1944 was, however, unusually high, but the north's bumper crop did not find its way south to Upper Egypt where there was no money to pay for it. Much of it was sold to Allied troops for hard currency. Times were prosperous for landowners and middlemen but not for the fellahin of Upper Egypt.

Reliable mortality statistics are not available for the 1942 and 1943 malaria epidemics. Most people did not willingly report deaths in their families.[59] Some simply felt that their sicknesses and deaths were not the business of the authorities. Births had often not been registered in the first place, and people were reluctant to face a penalty by reporting the deaths of nonregistered persons. An underpaid doctor would occasionally not sign a death certificate unless he was paid a sizable fee. In consequence people concealed their illnesses from government authorities and carried away the dead at night or hid them in baskets to bury them in secret. Furthermore, many of the malaria-stricken villages were remote and not connected with major towns by road, so it was difficult to report cases and deaths even if people were so inclined.[60] While provincial doctors were responsible for the systematic record keeping of infectious diseases, the *umda*s were supposed to report unusual incidence of disease or deaths to the authorities in Cairo. Because they were likely to be blamed for the bad health of their region, they understandably preferred to minimize problems. And, owing to the almost insurmountable difficulties of collecting them, vital statistics in remote regions were often not kept in the early 1940s. Ministry experts occasionally concocted case and death rates when the government insisted on having them.[61]

Estimates were therefore based on sketchy knowledge, which often varied according to political interest. The government tended to minimize mortality rates, while the opposition magnified them. For example, Khalil Abd al-Khaliq stated that there were 429,751 cases and 20,416 deaths from falciparum malaria in 1942 and 1943.[62] Tawfiq Shusha, permanent undersecretary of the Ministry of Health, in 1948 reported eleven thousand deaths from malaria in a report to the World Health Organization.[63] The palace and the opposition political parties claimed there had been one hundred thirty thousand deaths.[64] Colonel A. E. Richmond of the Royal Army Medical Corps gave one hundred eighty thousand as the best guess.[65] Alexander Kirk, U.S. minister in Cairo, reported to Washington, D.C., that there had been between one hundred thousand and two hundred thousand deaths from malaria.[66] J. Austin Kerr, a Rockefeller Foundation malaria expert, estimated that there had been 18,879 deaths and 188,947 cases in 1942 and 1943, but he noted that he had derived his figures from incomplete Ministry of Health statistics.[67] Asma Halim, a leftist journalist who had toured the malaria region in early 1944, reported that 94,155 people had perished.[68] The Ministry of Health data were derived from the number of officially recorded deaths from malaria, from the number of doses of Atabrine distributed, or from the increase in the number of deaths in 1942 and 1943 over the number of deaths in 1941.[69] The palace's estimate was based on a survey made by a royal commission.[70] The estimates by the British military, the American legation, and the journalist were apparently based on independent observation and rumor.

In October 1944 a British malaria expert made an analysis of the reported figures. He found 1,522 deaths from malaria had been officially reported in Qina and Aswan provinces but demonstrated that the case fatality rate was much higher in towns with medical officers, suggesting that reporting was more accurate there. He concluded that the epidemic was perhaps twice as severe as government figures indicated.[71]

Today the Ministry of Health estimates that one hundred thousand people perished in the malaria epidemic. It is possible to compare this figure against reported incidence rates. Unofficial reports indicated 50 to 99 percent incidence in Upper Egypt among a population of about 1.5 million. If incidence was 50 percent and the case fatality rate was about 10 percent, there might have been seven hundred fifty thousand cases and seventy-five thousand deaths. If incidence or fatalities were higher, mortality may well have reached the current ministry's estimate.

Mortality was high because of the poverty. As previously mentioned, many people, rich and poor, fell victim to malaria, but only the poor died. The malnourished were unable to resist the disease or to tolerate the antimalaria drugs, owing to their weakened condition. In some regions malaria was especially fatal to old people and to very young children.[72] Upper Egypt had long been impoverished, but during the war inflation had risen 130 percent, food and clothing supplies were scarce, and people were pushed below the subsistence level. Many people subsequently blamed the British army for buying up supplies that were needed in Upper Egypt.[73]

In December 1943 the Egyptian government began distributing free bread to the destitute to alleviate the severe malnutrition that made people vulnerable to malaria. Wakil announced to the press that the government had distributed bread to the poor and would sell flour and other foodstuffs at half price during the epidemic. It had sent teams of doctors, medical assistants, and malaria-control workers to the region. Teams had distributed medicines, spread Malariol over standing water, and sprayed trains, houses, and means of public transportation with pyrethrum insecticide.[74] Nevertheless, it was not enough. There were many reasons for the failure to control malaria, not all of them the fault of the ministry.

First, the scarcity of supplies had greatly complicated matters. The Ministry of Health had opted for Malariol rather than Paris green because it was easier to obtain and to use. Wartime conditions had hindered procurement of Paris green, while supplies of Malariol, composed of diesel oil and a spreading agent, were more readily available. Malariol could be sprayed by machine or by garden sprinkler; Paris green had to be carried to the site, then mixed with dirt or sand, and cast by hand. The reliance on Malariol meant that remote areas, accessible only by donkey or by foot, were left untreated. Malariol had other disadvantages: it was liable to theft because it could be used for fuel in cars and agricultural machinery; and the oil burned vegetation, so landowners were reluctant to use it.[75]

Second, the initial survey of gambiae spread was not accurate, and Ministry of Health authorities missed many foci. The ministry made a fundamental error by concentrating its control work on *birka* drainage. Eliminating all such water from the land was an impossible task and could not have eradicated *A. gambiae,* which preferred to breed in shallow irrigation canals or in seeping water found throughout Upper Egypt.

Third, mistakes were also made in management of the malaria service. Malaria workers were irregularly paid and were promoted on their connections rather than on merit. When a ministry malariologist reported that he had found *A. gambiae* in thirteen eradication zones, he received telegraphic orders from Abd al-Khaliq to fire immediately all thirteen of the men in whose zones gambiae had been found.[76] This order only encouraged workers not to report *A. gambiae* foci to the authorities. Men were often sent to the field with no training and told to get to work collecting gambiae larvae. About 40 percent of malaria workers contracted the disease. Often whole crews were unable to report for work of could work only briefly each day.[77] When malaria began spreading rapidly, the ministry in desperation shifted control workers from uninfected regions to malaria regions where they were to pass out Atabrine tablets. Then mosquitoes began breeding in the uninfected regions, and malaria soon appeared there as well.[78]

Fourth, physicians and nurses were in short supply. Often they had to be transferred from other services, which were not willing to give up their best staff members. So recent medical school graduates with no previous training in fieldwork were sent to Upper Egypt for one year. To fulfill their duties, they had to go by donkey to remote villages, but most of these workers rarely made such trips because they disliked the long hours and the difficult travel conditions.[79] Like other malaria workers, many physicians in infected regions contracted malaria. Doctors also disliked the service because it was far from Cairo, required field visits, and eliminated opportunities for private practice in Cairo.[80] The 50-percent pay increase and the promise of fellowships, missions abroad, and promotions did little to offset the antipathy. The government began forcing physicians to join the malaria treatment section and met with stiff resistance.[81] Nevertheless, many physicians, especially those in the Amiri hospitals in Isna, Luxor, and Aswan, served with great dedication despite their recurring attacks of malaria. Hospital nurses were few in number and were paid three pounds per month plus room and board, a low salary. There were, for example, only four nurses in the general hospital and three in the ophthalmic hospital in Luxor. While most nurses were men, these nurses were Muslim and Coptic women who had received their training in Cairo. All of these nurses tended male and female patients of both faiths.[82]

Fifth, the underpaid "*sahha*" (a slang expression for Ministry of Health officials) were not entirely incorruptible. Persons could avoid having their houses disinfected (with a smelly cresol compound) by buying off the *sahha*. The *sahha* sometimes grabbed people's wrists and announced that they felt feverish. The victims would be taken to the infectious diseases section of the local hospital unless a certain sum of money could be paid.[83] Hamed Ammar recalled that, during the 1943 malaria epidemic, the inhabitants of Silwa, a town in Aswan province, came to distrust the recently built health center not only because it was built near the cemetery, which was a bad omen, but because in Silwa (as elsewhere) dying away from one's relatives and home was considered the worst thing that could happen to anyone.[84]

Sixth, environmental conditions made control work exceedingly difficult. The mosquito larvae could be found in the smallest pools of standing water throughout the region. Roads were few, and control workers had to travel long distances on foot or on donkey. Dwellings offered excellent habitats for the adult mosquitoes, which preferred warm, dark places. A malaria worker described the interior of a house in Badari in which an adult gambiae mosquito had been collected: "one water buffalo; about ten goats and kids, numerous pigeons sitting on eggs in holes in the walls—and also a large family. When asked about where they slept, they pointed to the floor in the corridor of the house. . . . Cornstalk thatch is the most common roofing material, because of the scarcity of beams to hold up bricks, which might otherwise be used. Such houses are very difficult to flit [spray with insecticide]."[85]

Despite the many difficulties of the antimalaria campaign, Wakil put things in their best light, at least for public consumption. On 13 October 1943, after touring Upper Egypt, he announced that the outbreak was very limited and that the ban on travel to Luxor and Aswan would be lifted in the winter.[86] In a major address given at the Wafd party's silver jubilee celebration in November 1943, Wakil said that, while medicine and public health had advanced slowly in Egypt in comparison with countries in the West, Egypt was successfully combating the epidemic in the interior by modern scientific methods. He then said that health conditions in Egypt had worsened in the twentieth century for four reasons: decline in the income of the majority, lack of public education and 80 percent illiteracy, lack of adequate funds for health improvement, and absence of a health program.[87] Wakil did not mention the British or Egyptian public-health policies of this era, the shift in irrigation methods, the Great Depression, or other internal and international causes. His four reasons were designed to support the Wafdist political platform.

Wakil announced that the 1943–44 budget of the Ministry of Health was £E 4.5 million, the largest ever, and that £E 2.5 million were to be allocated for the village health centers in 1944. Each province was to have several such centers designed to serve twenty-five thousand people or more. He then outlined other plans, including fighting endemic diseases; expanding clean water supplies; and building new hospitals, isolation centers for those with tuberculosis and leprosy, and schools for physicians, midwives, technicians, and pharmacists.[88] In December 1943 at the height of the epidemic, the ministry issued a press release entitled "Success for the Hunters of Gambiae."[89] In the release Wakil announced that the situation was better than it had been in 1942 because of the ministry's actions. He assured the public that the ministry had the situation in hand.[90] In an article entitled "Most Important Incidents of 1943," published in *al-Ahram* the last day of the year, the malaria epidemic was not included. The article cited only the military order of

20 January 1943, which called for filling the *birka*s.[91] The government had valiantly attempted to deal with the malaria crisis, had done its best to reassure the public that all was well, but could not conceal the magnitude of the outbreak for long.

In December many people in Cairo who owned land in Upper Egypt traveled there on holiday and witnessed the conditions firsthand. Nubians who worked in the homes of the wealthy in Cairo told their employers about the deaths of their relatives from malaria. Soon rumors of a disaster in Upper Egypt began spreading through the city.

3

Elite Women and King Faruq to the Rescue

The malaria story broke early in January 1944, when Princess Chevikar (Shiyuwihkar), one of the leaders of Cairo society, called a press conference at her palace to announce an unprecedented relief project.[1] Princess Chevikar was head of the women's section of the Mabarra Muhammad Ali (or the Mabarra). Her husband, Ilhami Husayn Pasha, was titular head of the Mabarra. She had been briefly married to her cousin Ahmad Fuad before he became king of Egypt and before Faruq was born. The marriage ended badly, but Chevikar had reestablished herself in a position she might have held had she become queen. During Faruq's reign, she held elegant receptions that the king often attended. She also presided over the Mabarra's fund-raising events.

At the press conference, Princess Chevikar told the assembled journalists that one of the women in the Mabarra Muhammad Ali had just returned from a visit to Upper Egypt, where she had learned of the malaria disaster. The situation there was grave: she thought it was time for the government to stop making long speeches and to tell the truth about it. She had quickly contacted members of the Mabarra, who in turn began organizing a relief mission for the victims of malaria composed of the volunteers, two doctors, and two nurses. The mission would go to the malaria region, where it would distribute clothes, blankets, food, and medicines free of charge to the needy. She assured the press that the minister of health had given the women permission to work in the region, and she added that the women's motives were humanitarian and that everyone should support them. She concluded the press conference by asking the public to donate money to the organization and to support its efforts.[1]

Behind the scenes, Hidiya Afifi Barakat (1899–1969), the moving force of the Mabarra, was organizing the teams of women, collecting funds for supplies, and mobilizing support for their mission. Barakat was one of the pioneers of the Egyptian feminist movement and had been active in the nationalistic movement of 1919. In the 1920s and 1930s she had organized girls' schools, nursing schools, homes for the aged, and special-care facilities for babies, in addition to the clinics and hospitals of the Mabarra Muhammad Ali. Now, with the news of the malaria epidemic, she turned her attention organizing the Mabarra's new relief mission.

The Women's Committee of the Red Crescent Association also met and planned a similar relief operation. It obtained permission from the Ministry of Health to work in Isna, a town in Upper Egypt. On 17 January 1944 the undersecretary of the Ministry of Health met with representatives of the Mabarra and the Red Crescent to set guidelines for their activities. Abd al-Wahid al-Wakil announced that he would depart for the region in a week to check on their work. Two days later, on 19 January, the Mabarra Muhammad Ali mission departed for Luxor. The women traveled in a railway car loaded with food, medicine, and clothes. In the party were Amina Sidqi, daughter of Ismail Sidqi, a former prime minister and prominent economist who advocated industrial development in Egypt; Firdaws Shitta, a member of a prominent landowning family; and Mary Kahil, who throughout her long life (1889–1979) was one of Egypt's most noted philanthropists. The Mabarra doctor, Dr. Binyamin, and its nurses, Abla Sa'id Ahmad and Ni'matullah Amin, were responsible for medical care.

Meanwhile, the Red Crescent women prepared their mission by collecting *galabiyas* (garments worn by men and women) for distribution.[3] Safiyya Zaghlul, widow of Sa'd Zaghlul, founder of the Wafd party and leader of the nationalist movement following World War I, went to the Red Crescent hospital on Queen Nazli Street to inspect preparations for the project. Zaghlul's grandnephew, Mustafa Amin, editor of *Ithnayn wa Dunya*, a propalace weekly magazine, ran a cover story on the women (fig. 2).[4] On 22 January 1944 the Red Crescent mission departed

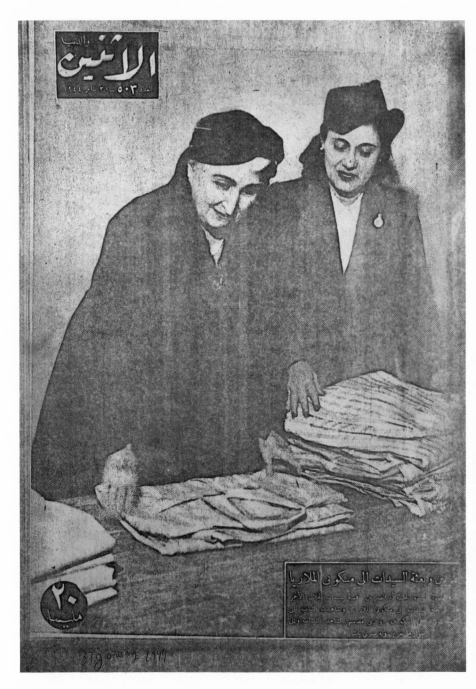

Fig. 2. Safiyya Zaghlul (left) and Nahid Sirri (right) inspecting *galabiya*s being prepared for shipment to Upper Egypt. Source: *Ithnayn wa Dunya*, 21 January 1944.

Cairo for Isna. Four women were in the first party: Nahid Sirri, wife of Husayn Sirri, the former prime minister; Lutfiya Yusri, Chevikar's daughter and wife of Ahmad Hasanayn, chief of the royal cabinet; Gertrude Butrus Ghali, Swiss wife of Mirit Butrus Ghali, a leader of the Coptic community; and Layla Shawarbi, daughter of Muhammad Shawarbi and sister of Abd al-Hamid Shawarbi, both prominent land-owners and political figures. Other members later participated, rotating in shifts or organizing support work in Cairo.[5] Muhammad Shahin, personal physician to Faruq and the Royal Palace, assisted and often accompanied the women.

Most of the volunteers in both the Red Crescent and the Mabarra Muhammad Ali were from prominent political families associated with the palace. Few had connections to the Wafd party. The women were Muslim, Christian, and Jewish; most were wealthy; many were educated in French convents and had participated in charitable work in Cairo. They had learned skills that they could not use in gainful employment because it was not acceptable for elite women at the time.

Forty years later Abla Sa'id Ahmad, one of the Mabarra nurses, re-called that in Luxor the Mabarra rented a house with a large garden. The women visited villages around the town and worked out a system of ration cards. They distributed beans, barley, vegetables, fruit, and iron pills. Thousands of ration cards were distributed to men, women, and children. The nurse remembered that they all worked twenty out of twenty-four hours a day. The volunteer women themselves were not medically qualified and performed only minor first aid. While making their rounds, they referred patients to the medical staff or, in severe cases, arranged their transport to the hospital. Within days the Mabarra had set up a soup kitchen, which fed two thousand people per day. The women organized trucks and camel caravans to distribute food to six thousand families living in outlying villages per week. Mary Kahil had truckloads of rice and wheat delivered to Upper Egypt at her own expense.[6] The women found that the inhabitants of the malaria-stricken regions themselves were generally responsive to them and admitted them into their homes more readily than they admitted government officials.[7]

Ithnayn wa Dunya sent a journalist to Luxor to report on the activities of the Mabarra Muhammad Ali mission. He was taken about by

Amina Sidqi, who was making a survey of the needs of malaria victims for food, clothing, and medication. He found Firdaws Shitta managing the group's finances, while Mary Kahil was making house calls with the Mabarra's nurses to supervise the distribution of rations. When he finished his tour, the reporter went with the women to the popular kitchen. There he found a senator from the region, Mahmud Muhasib, helping to hand out bread, vegetables, and fruit to the people.[8] In his report, the journalist emphasized the dedication of the women and the magnitude of the work they were carrying out.

Meanwhile, the Red Crescent women had organized their distribution center at Isna, where they stayed at the rest house of the sugar factory. Once established, the women began making rounds in the surrounding villages. Gertrude Butrus Ghali, who had gone to Isna with the first group, kept a diary in which she described how the women went house-to-house to see if there was malaria or deprivation within. She wrote that in some houses whole families lay upon the ground too weak to work in the fields or even to move. The people were like living skeletons; their clothes were in rags. Some shook from malaria fever.[9] The Red Crescent women found the people lacked both clothes and blankets and had no protection from the bitter cold of winter. Some families had Atabrine tablets, but many people were too weak from hunger to tolerate the medicine. To facilitate the dispensing of relief, the women made a survey of each house, listing the number of inhabitants and their need for medicine, food, clothing, and blankets. Then they gave the families ration cards that enabled one member to collect a week's supplies from the distribution center in Isna. The women made notes of the more severe cases so that the treatment service could take them to a hospital.[10] Gertrude Ghali recalls that she and one of her colleagues led a camel caravan to stricken villages when the camel driver did not appear one morning. She retains a photograph of the expedition showing the two women leading the caravan, one on a horse and the other, who could not ride, on a donkey. Within a month the Red Crescent women had hired and were supervising a staff that prepared and dispensed meals to forty-three hundred people per day in Isna's open-air cinema. The Red Crescent usually had five to ten members working in Upper Egypt at one time. Most stayed in shifts of one or one and one-half months. The Red Crescent later expanded additional centers in Kom Ombo, Matana, and elsewhere.

Jemima Abbud, the British wife of the famous entrepreneur and industrialist Ahmad Abbud, had set up a soup kitchen on her husband's sugarcane estates in Armant in December 1943, when his sugar company was losing its workers to the famine and to malaria. Asma Halim, the leftist journalist, visited the Armant Sugar Company in late February 1944. She found that many of the workers were emaciated and had yellow faces and eyes, indicating that they were still suffering from malaria. One man said he had been sick for one hundred days but had stayed at home for only forty-five. Since his wife was also sick and unable to care for the children, he returned home each evening to feed them bread, *tamiyya* (fried cake made of ground bean stalk flour), and lettuce. In the morning and at noon his family ate only bread. He said the company distributed bread, lentils, and beans to the workers every day but only at noon. Because the workers worked only half of the month at night, they had this factory meal only half of the month.[11] Jemima Abbud later joined the Red Crescent, which had opened a food distribution center in Armant. At Luxor, Halim visited the Mabarra soup kitchen where she found lines of men, women, and children, each with a plate and a utensil. In between the two large pots of food were police, women of the Mabarra, and members of the Senate and Chamber of Deputies. A photographer was taking pictures while a senator, whose sister was in the Mabarra, distributed oranges to the people. When the photographer left, the senator tossed the oranges back into the basket, nodded to his sister, and departed.[12] Others shared Halim's opinion that some of the politicians who associated themselves with the woman were more interested in political advantage than in public service.

From the start Wafdist officials recognized that the women's activities put them in a bad light because the women's efforts implied that the Wafd had failed to deal with the malaria disaster. The government was therefore anxious to demonstrate that it was leading the battle against malaria. Upon first news of the women's plans, Ahmad Hamza, the minister of supplies, had announced to the press that the government would supply the women with cereals, sugar, oil, and clothing to dispense. He went to Upper Egypt in February to check on the women's work and assured the public that the government had never failed to come to the aid of the sick (fig. 3).[13]

After the women had been working for ten days, Chevikar called a second press conference. She told the press assembled in her palace that

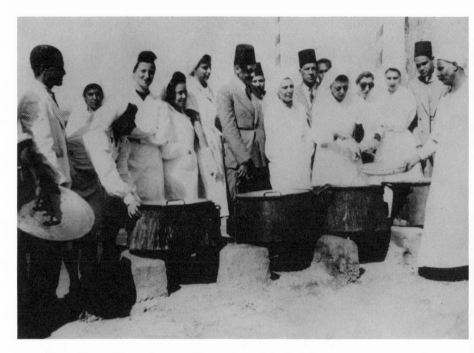

Fig. 3. Ahmad Hamza (center) with members of the Red Crescent at soup kitchen in Isna, February 1944. Courtesy of Gertrude Hoffman Ghali.

the first report from the mission indicated that the people were very sick and that mortality had been exceptionally high for the past two years. Some families had vanished, while those fellahin who survived were not able to work for lack of food. She urged the press to make the country conscious of the disaster. If nothing were done to fight the epidemic, the number of cases would double the following winter, and the fellahin would be unable to work. Eventually, if malaria spread, Egypt's land would have to be abandoned. She said the minister of health had visited the Mabarra headquarters in Luxor as planned and had praised the activities of the women. She asked the reporters to write something every day in their newspapers; to ask people to donate money, products, clothing, or medicine; and to attend a concert the Mabarra was holding to raise money for the poor in Qina and Aswan.[14]

The women acquired most of their funds through such public appeals. In addition, the American Red Cross donated one thousand blankets and one thousand doses of quinine (fifteen thousand tablets). The women also asked for two mobile canteen units for food distribution from the American army; but the American Red Cross representative recommended against U.S. Army participation in food distribution because he thought the Red Crescent society had purchased enough supplies to last through the emergency, which he optimistically thought would continue only about ten more weeks.[15]

The women's missions had been enormously successful in drawing public attention to the crisis. They had also indirectly suggested that the Wafd government had not satisfactorily dealt with the emergency. This situation presented the palace with a golden opportunity.

The first week of February 1944, Killearn noticed that Faruq was in an exceptionally good mood.[16] He was right: the king had decided to spend his twenty-fourth birthday, a public holiday, inspecting the stricken regions and visiting the women's missions in Isna and Luxor. He would thereby demonstrate his concern for the victims of famine and malaria, show support for the women's missions, gain favorable publicity by associating with them, and signal that the Wafd government had neglected its responsibilities. This action might force the palace to take charge.

On 7 February the king received Mustafa Nahhas but said nothing about the plan he and his advisors had worked out. On 9 February Ahmad Hassanein, the chief of the royal cabinet and husband of Lutfiya Yusri, Princess Chevikar's daughter who was working with the Red Crescent, simply contacted the ministers of the interior and health informing them that the king was departing to visit the sick and starving in the infected provinces.[17]

On the morning of 10 February the king left Cairo quietly by special train accompanied by Ahmad Hassanein and three of the leading propalace journalists, among whom was Mustafa Amin.[18] That day there was not a word in the newspapers, but "as the glittering white royal diesel train sped up country . . . , the news seemed to spread ahead of it like wildfire."[19]

On 11 February the nation awakened to the news that the king had left Cairo to spend his birthday in the malaria-stricken region of Upper Egypt. This year while the nation celebrated the day with visits and feasts, the king was away from Cairo. Faruq spent two days in Qina and Aswan, where he visited the headquarters of the Mabarra Muhammad Ali and the Red Crescent and toured the region. He announced that he had gone to Upper Egypt to see conditions for himself because he knew the people had faith in him.[20]

The propalace journals were full of photographs of the king inspecting the Mabarra Muhammad Ali food distribution center in Luxor, posing with women from the Red Crescent and the Mabarra, and attending a banquet in his honor. Faruq announced that he was very proud of the Egyptian women who had sacrificed their own welfare for the sake of the poor. There were photographs of Faruq visiting a hut, flanked by Ahmad Hasanayn, Karim Thabit, and other palace officials. *Al-Musawwar,* a propalace weekly magazine, published photographs of the king's luncheon in Luxor with Amina Sidqi, Mary Kahil, Firdaws Shitta, Ni'matullah Amin, and the palace officials.[21] Faruq prayed in the Isna mosque, having given instructions that rich and poor alike be admitted with him. *Ruz al-Yusuf* reported that such news was never published. Whatever the king touched was purchased by a member of his retinue, and so a piece of bread was purchased for £E 100 and a can of honey also for £E 100. The magazine called the visit a "veritable dream."[22]

Faruq donated £E 10,000 to the Mabarra Muhammad Ali and Red Crescent societies and issued a public appeal for increased donations. Donations poured in. Parliament passed a recommendation to allocate funds to assist. The foreign community also contributed, often through the Red Crescent, which was associated with the International Red Cross. The Red Crescent volunteers appealed for empty bottles to be used for the distribution of medicine. Readers of *al-Ahram* donated £E 871 and 448 milliemes. Charitable societies with foreign memberships abandoned plans to collect for war victims abroad and collected for the malaria victims in Egypt instead. The government of Lebanon donated L£ 95,000. Officers in the British army collected and donated twenty thousand articles of clothing for the poor in the area.[23] The U.S. Air Force donated blankets and other supplies to the Red Crescent (fig. 4).

Newspaper coverage, of course, reflected the political tendency of each newspaper. As seen above, the propalace journals, such as *Ruz al-Yusuf, Ithnayn wa Dunya,* and *Akhir Sa'a,* which the palace supported

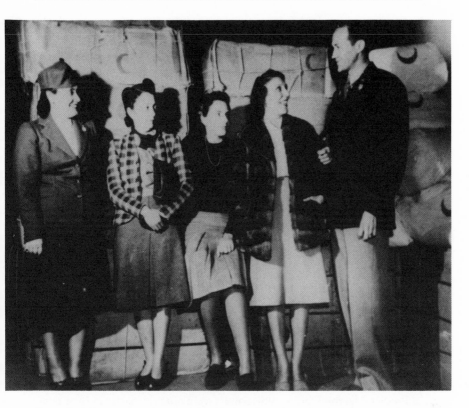

Fig. 4. Red Crescent members receiving blankets from the U.S. Air Force. Photograph taken in Cairo, 1944. Courtesy of Gertrude Hoffman Ghali.

financially, were generally enthusiastic in their coverage of the missions. Such journals predictably rhapsodized about the formerly secluded women who had left their luxurious palaces and pleasant pastimes for a hard life in Upper Egypt and congratulated the king on his birthday visit. But at least one article in the propalace press was highly critical.

In her effort to gain favorable publicity, Chevikar had asked Ihsan Abd al-Qadus, son of Fatima al-Yusuf, the founder of *Ruz al-Yusuf,* and later one of Egypt's prominent authors, to go to Upper Egypt to cover the women's activities. Abd al-Qadus, who was then in his early twenties, did so and reported that the women were from the class whose members were the real mosquitoes who "suck the peoples blood and turn it into cakes, caviar, and champagne."[24] Their class was, he said, the real epidemic that had entered villages, alleys, and houses and ravaged the people. The palaces of the rich, he stated, were no better than the pools of water in which the mosquitoes bred. He said the number of women working in Upper Egypt could be counted on the fingers of one hand. M. M. Afifi, Chevikar's secretary, had told him that the Mabarra had need of volunteers, but the elite women refused to volunteer because they might miss the film starring Robert Taylor, the sales at the Cicurel, Umar Effendi, and Benzion department stores, or a dancing party at L'Auberge des Pyramides. The women could not pull themselves away from their mirrors, perfume, powder boxes, and makeup. Meanwhile, death was reflected in mirrors in Upper Egypt, where the miserable conditions put a new yellow and blue makeup on the faces of the disease's victims. He concluded that people had to take a stand to remake society from its foundations.[25] Chevikar was presumably most displeased with the article.

Such views were rarely expressed in print during the war because the journals in which they were usually found were banned.[26] *Ruz al-Yusuf* alone occasionally published such views as those of Asma Halim and Abd al-Qadus because it specialized in pointed political commentary and satire while maintaining a fundamentally propalace stance.

Predictably, the Wafdist newspapers were unenthusiastic in their coverage of the women's missions and scarcely mentioned the king's visit. The slightly pro-Wafd *Progres egyptien* ran a series on the women just after they began work, but the series featured an interview with Wakil, who was checking on the women's work. Wakil, who only referred to the volunteers in passing, told the *Progres* reporter that he had a five-year plan for public health reform after the war and that providence had perhaps sent the epidemic so that Egypt would awaken to the terrible misery of the fellah.[27] *Al-Misri,* the official Wafd daily newspaper, provided extensive coverage of Wafd government projects but did not cover the women's missions or Faruq's trip. The day after the king's birthday, the paper published a prepared statement saying only that the nation joined the king in celebrating the event and that governmental officials had called at the palace to offer their best wishes.[28] The Wafd government thus signaled its displeasure at being upstaged in this manner.

Conservative Muslim groups disapproved of the women, who were mostly French educated and Western in their behavior and dress, and accused them of merely seeking publicity for themselves.[29] But public opinion in Egypt's foreign communities was generally favorable. A typical letter to the editor was published in the pro-French *La bourse egyptienne*. It praised the simple patriotism of the Red Crescent women as they departed by train dressed in their blue uniforms. It said that the women were very conscious of the difficulties they would have to surmount but that they were anxious to do their best to help their compatriots.[30] The foreign communities were accustomed to women organizing such philanthropic services in their own societies and approved of it in Egypt.

Faruq returned to Cairo 14 February 1944 to an enthusiastic reception. A special Friday *khutbah* (sermon), praising the women and the king, was read to the king, the prime minister, and the members of the government assembled at the Sultan Hasan mosque and in mosques throughout Egypt. The imam (prayer leader) said that there was no one in Egypt who had not heard the cries of pain from the sick and the poor of Qina and Aswan; from the people who had built the canals, the barrages, the bridges, and the roads of Egypt; and who manned the factories and the mines. Poverty had bitten the people with its teeth, and sickness had spent their bodies. Orphans and widows were everywhere. Houses were silent and graves were full. The noble-hearted women of the Mabarra Muhammad Ali and the Red Crescent were the first to leave their families and their children and to hasten to bring clothing, food, blankets, and medicine to the destitute. They alone, he said, were not afraid of death.[31]

The imam asked if it was dignified for men to sit back while others volunteered to help. He said the king had set a good example by going to comfort the sick and the poor in their huts and shacks, to see for himself, and to understand their problems. The examples set by the women and their king should encourage people to double their efforts and to give generously.[32]

The *khutbah*, clearly prepared by propalace religious authorities, made no mention of the Wafd government's efforts to cope with the malaria epidemic and implied that the women and the king were the first to take action against the disaster. The *khutbah* was a direct attack on the government. Furthermore, the king had gone to Upper Egypt without checking with the government. He had taken no ministers with him, only the royal entourage and prominent propalace journalists. He had officially received only the women of the Mabarra and the Red Crescent and none of the local Wafd party officials.

Toward the end of February, Prince Muhammad Ali, the elderly heir to the throne and a strong supporter of the British, informed the British embassy that "the Royal Entourage were set on making political capital out of the situation in Upper Egypt" and that Princess Chevikar had telephoned one of the princesses in Cairo to say that King Faruq should dismiss the Mustafa Nahhas government while he had the Wafd at his mercy.[33] Faruq was hoping to do just that.

Nahhas tried to counter the anti-Wafdist publicity generated by the women's missions and the king's birthday visit by granting an interview to *Akhir Sa'a,* a glossy propalace magazine. In a slap at the women's relief missions, he asserted that the government had been distributing food and medicine long before the arrival of "those who praise their own efforts while saying nothing had been done."[34] He added that people who cared for humanity and charity should not glorify themselves by exaggerating the misery of those in need. The government, he insisted, had directed the Mabarra and Red Crescent to the region, had organized their work, and had given them supplies.[35] The *Egyptian Gazette,* mouthpiece of the British embassy and pro-Wafd at the time, gave limited coverage to the women's missions. The newspaper carried Chevikar's appeals for donations and sent a reporter to Isna to accompany Red Crescent women on their rounds, but after describing the disaster he merely emphasized the limited scale of the women's work.[36]

The women were well aware of the controversy their activities elicited. Nahid Sirri, for example, sidestepped pointed questions in an interview published in *Ruz al-Yusuf.* She was spending a few days in Cairo and was about to return to the Red Crescent mission in Isna. She told the reporter that she had worked for the Red Crescent for more than three years, but she had never seen such a disaster as that in Qina and Aswan. She had recently read in some newspapers that the Red Crescent had gone there not to save the poor but just to create propaganda. She replied that it was a pity to have such things said at a time when the Red Crescent's work was needed. The reporter asked her about the problem of poverty and disease. She replied that she could not express an opinion about the problem because she had not studied it and that the women's mission was only to give aid to the victims.[37] This comment suggests that she preferred to avoid such politically sensitive questions as the role of the wealthy landowners (her social class) in the impoverishment of the fellahin.

Were the women mere tools of the palace? While the missions had temporarily enabled the palace to win a measure of public appreciation for its concern for the victims of famine and malaria and while the missions increased the women's awareness of the distress existing outside their social class, they also won a new and expanded role for women in public service.

The missions were unprecedented because, while neither visiting female nurses (*hakimas*) nor women philanthropists were a new phenomenon in Egypt, neither customarily traveled long distances to establish and administer large-scale relief programs by themselves. The *hakimas* had worked for the government health service under the direction of government officials.[38] Women philanthropists before the twentieth century had usually carried out their charitable work from within their homes with the assistance of male intermediaries, who represented them in official arrangements. In the first decades of the twentieth century, the Mabarra women had confined themselves to raising funds and managing their dispensaries and clinics. During the bombing of Alexandria in 1940 and 1941, the volunteers had organized soup kitchens and shelters for those who had sought refuge in Cairo. During the malaria epidemic, the women of the Mabarra and the Red Crescent traveled independently of their families to organize their own large-scale relief programs and sought to draw attention to their efforts to gain public support. This activity was unprecedented and accounted in large part for the impression that they made on public opinion.[39]

Should they then be considered feminists? Nawal El Saadawi, the prominent Egyptian feminist writer, has argued that, by the 1940s, "the women's movement [had] become a pawn utilized to serve the interests of the palace and the reactionary parties. It kept away from active involvement in national and political life of the country and limited its activities to charitable and social welfare work."[40] This statement is misleading because it equates the women's or feminist movement with the volunteers. Only a few of the volunteer women, including Hidiya Barakat, Mary Kahil, Amina Sidqi, Nahid Sirri, and Firdaws Shitta, had participated in the feminist movement.

Huda Sha'rawi (1879–1947), who had founded the Egyptian Feminist Union in 1923, did not participate in the missions. Sha'rawi was by far the most prominent Egyptian woman of her generation. She was known for her long association with the Wafd party—an association that was largely terminated in the 1940s—for her anti-British sentiments, for her participation in nationalistic struggles, and for her organizing on behalf of Egyptian women. Sha'rawi had been one of the founding members of the Mabarra Muhammad Ali in 1909 and was an honorary member of the Red Crescent, but she was not active in either organization in the 1940s. While the women worked in Upper Egypt, she was organizing the Second Congress for Arab Women, which was to be held in Cairo in December 1944.[41]

The membership of the Egyptian Feminist Union and the voluntary organizations were largely drawn from the wealthy classes and a few women were active in both, but the goals of the groups differed considerably. Although they did have at one time a Committee for Health Affairs of Women and Children and a dispensary among their other social services, the feminists concentrated on eliminating the subordinate status of women in society, while the volunteers focused on the provisioning of public health and welfare services to the needy. The women's charitable and social welfare activities, though they afforded the participants unprecedented experience in public life, should therefore be considered separately from the organized feminist movement.

In recent years, sociologists studying upper-class women's voluntary associations in Western countries have concluded that their basic motivation has been class maintenance: the women seek to justify their privileges and status by performing good works for society.[42] While some of the Egyptian women may have had such concerns and while others may have primarily enjoyed the publicity or the unaccustomed adventure, most were hoping to use their skills to help others. In other words, among the complex motives that included desire for class maintenance, support for palace interests, increased women's participation in public life, and enjoyment of adventure and publicity, most important was the desire for public service. Or as Wadud Fayzi Musa, one of the Mabarra volunteers, put it when interviewed in 1986, "we wanted to do something for our country."[43]

Interviewed forty years later, Mustafa Amin, the formerly propalace journalist, now a prominent newspaper editor, praised the volunteer women's sincerity and dedication and was most anxious that their story be told. He thought that the most important result was that the women in the Mabarra and Red Crescent had seen for themselves the differences between the rich and the underdogs of society.[44] This recognition of the extent of impoverishment led the volunteers to expand their existing relief and medical assistance programs rather than to engage in political reform.

The women had aided a substantial number of the victims of famine and malaria. They had intentionally drawn public attention to the emergency in Upper Egypt. This attention had given King Faruq a chance to go to the rescue himself. The resulting publicity had heated up the power struggle between the palace, the Wafd, and the British and now set in motion an enormous political controversy. In the spring of 1943 malaria became a potent political weapon.

4

Malaria in Politics

The palace, the Wafd, and the British embassy had been dueling with one another since Egypt had become nominally independent. Now each sought to blame another for the malaria epidemic and to exonerate itself. The resulting controversy showed that public health had become an issue that could threaten governmental longevity.

While Faruq was on his birthday visit to the malaria-stricken regions of Upper Egypt, Killearn had reported to the foreign office that the government had still not accepted British military assistance in dealing with the malaria epidemic. He had, however, "put some more ginger in two nights ago. Things move with exasperating slowness in this country."[1] He was exasperated because since the end of December 1943 he had been urging the Wafd government to accept British assistance. At that time he had told British army authorities that he thought that, if the Egyptians were left to their own devices, they would continue to assure the public that all was well until the nation faced a serious epidemic in Upper Egypt and in Lower Egypt.[2] Killearn had become alarmed by a British military report on the malaria situation. The report had said that the situation had become critical because of (1) the risk to British troops; (2) the magnitude of sickness and death among laborers in agriculture, sugar production, and other industries that were needed for the war effort; (3) the threat to Lower Egypt; (4) the heavy consumption of antimalarial drugs, which were in short supply throughout the world; and (5) the unnecessary suffering in Upper Egypt. Measures being undertaken by the Egyptian government were, the report said, inadequate, and *A. gambiae* had been found near Asiut, indicating that it was still spreading downriver. The report urged the Egyptian government to accept British proposals for malaria-control work.[3]

Under pressure, the Egyptian Minister of Health had formed a General Health Committee consisting of four Egyptians, two British, and two Americans. The British embassy and the American legation agreed to have an unpublicized committee between themselves to prevent the Egyptians from playing one off against the other. It was an arrangement tried earlier by the cereals board, which had "cut down on acrimonious correspondence between the two sides."[4] The suspicions between the British and Americans, however, remained acute.

Upon Faruq's return to Cairo, Killearn telegraphed the foreign office to say that the king had gained "well-merited kudos" for his inspection of conditions in Upper Egypt.[5] He lamented that the government had been "culpably negligent and dilatory" in dealing with the malaria epidemic.[6] He concluded that the king had every right to take matters into his own hands and to take the initiative in helping his suffering subjects.[7] Thoroughly irritated, he rang up Amin Osman, the minister of finance and the liaison between the British embassy and the Wafd government, and told him that the government was "missing the bus" and that it had been six weeks since the British had presented their plan for dealing with the malaria epidemic.[8] The next day he told Osman that Faruq had stolen the government's thunder and that he foresaw a "pretty violent political reaction throughout the country."[9] British experts, he said, had given the government a plan for an antimalarial campaign six weeks before and had been put off.[10] The Wafd had played into the hands of King Faruq.

Finally, Wakil agreed to accept the assistance of three malaria-control units seconded from the British army that would, he said tersely, be added to the one hundred Egyptian malaria-control units already at work, whereupon he proceeded to drag his feet on implementing the agreement.[11] He then announced a plan to raise taxes and enlist the help of the Egyptian army in fighting malaria. He said that he would ask Parliament to allocate £E 1.0 million for food subsidies, £E 0.3 million for clothing, and £E 0.2 million for medicines. Funds were to be raised by an additional "epidemic tax" on landowners in Upper Egypt, a measure that had been submitted to Parliament on 6 January

1944. Those paying less than ten pounds per year in taxes were to be exempted, those paying more would have their taxes raised in proportion to their incomes. On 11 February while the king was on his birthday tour of the malaria-stricken region, the Wafd government had announced the new law calling for an additional tax on the provinces of Qina and Aswan, and that the Egyptian army would be sent to distribute food and to provide transportation for control workers.[12] The Wafd party was strong in Upper Egypt, where it was supported by many of the wealthier landowners, and the government was confident the tax would be accepted. The malaria crisis, however, had passed the stage of easy resolution.

In January 1944 Faruq had charged that the Wafd government was allowing sales of wheat from Lower Egypt and cloth from the Bank Misr's Mahalla al-Kubra textile factories to the British army while the fellahin were starving and facing the winter nearly naked. At that time Amin Osman had assured Killearn that the charges were groundless and that there was plenty of food in the country. The problem, Osman had said, was faulty distribution for which the British, and especially the British army, were in no sense responsible.[13] A few hours after he returned to Cairo, Faruq called in the prime minister and the ministers of health, social affairs, public works, interior, supplies, and *waqfs*. He told them that they had failed to deal with the situation and that food and medicine being sent to Upper Egypt had not reached the population. Ahmad Hamza, the minister of supplies, replied to Faruq that there was no shortage of cereals in Egypt but acknowledged that the Mahalla al-Kubra company had sold cloth to the British army. Wakil added that the problem was not malaria or British military purchases but malnutrition. The malnutrition, he said, was caused by the landowners who had not paid their workers or fellahin enough to feed and clothe themselves. This charge indirectly implicated the king who owned large estates in Upper Egypt.[14] The palace and the Wafd government had now declared war against each other.[15]

Faruq continued to insist that the British army had sequestered food that was needed by the fellahin, thus causing the starvation that had exacerbated the epidemic. To Killearn's aggravation, Faruq passed the rumor on to the wife of the Soviet minister at a dinner party. Killearn was even more aggravated by Wakil, who was spreading a rumor that the British had offered their medical advice simply to gain control of parts of the Egyptian government.[16]

Killearn faced a dilemma. The British had installed the Wafd government by force. The war was still underway, and Killearn depended upon the Wafd to support the Allied war effort. Yet malaria was still spreading and could also endanger the Allied war effort. The Wafd was not coping with the epidemic and was blaming it on the British. He decided to counterattack.

First, he published a lead article in the *Egyptian Gazette,* mouthpiece of the British embassy. The article said that the government should take action on a large scale to deal with the malaria epidemic and that distribution of food and medicine was necessary but not sufficient. Mosquitoes were continuing to spread, and if they reached the Delta, Egypt was doomed. The article concluded that the benevolent societies did not have the resources to stamp out the epidemic.[17] This article was intended to serve as a warning to the Wafd government: action against the malaria epidemic was needed immediately if British support was to continue.

Second, he issued a communiqué to be published in the Arabic- and foreign-language presses. The communiqué said that the situation in Upper Egypt was not due to a shortage of food in the country, that large quantities of wheat from the 1943 harvest remained available to the Egyptian government, and that food supplies were more than adequate to meet the needs of the country until the next harvest. The communiqué concluded, *"If local shortages occur, these can only be due to failures in the system of distribution for which the British authorities are not responsible"* (emphasis in original).[18] Fuad Sirag al-Din, minister of the interior and deputy chief of the Wafd party, insisted that the italicized sentence be censored before being published.[19]

Third, the British embassy published the entire communiqué in the *Egyptian Gazette.* Sirag al-Din protested to the British embassy against the publication of a censored item in the newspaper.[20] Killearn protested that the Egyptian government had tampered with an official British statement. Mustafa Amin, the propalace journalist, then asked Killearn if there was any objection to his publishing the entire statement. Killearn remarked that this communiqué was of interest only because Amin was becoming the "running dog" of the palace.[21] Killearn suspected that the palace was encouraging the dispute. The censorship controversy was resolved when Killearn agreed to withdraw his protest on condition that the government not censor future British embassy communiqués.[22]

Fourth, Killearn issued a second communiqué, which was published in the *Egyptian Gazette* on 27 February. This communiqué said that British and American army experts had repeatedly offered to help deal with the malaria epidemic but that their offers had not been accepted. Now the British army was offering to send two malaria-control units and a field laboratory to Upper Egypt. British and American authorities had made available to the Egyptian government large supplies of Atabrine, Paris green, and pyrethrum spray.[23] Killearn anticipated a strong reaction from Nahhas over the second communiqué.[24]

At the end of February, Nahhas and Killearn met. Nahhas told Killearn that he was up to his neck in difficulties and was ready to resign if there were serious differences between the British and the Wafd government. Nevertheless, Nahhas thought he could still do "good work for the Ally and the war effort."[25] Killearn replied that the British would continue to support the Wafd government.[26]

The next skirmish was to take place in the Chamber of Deputies of the Egyptian Parliament. While the malaria crisis was brewing, two opposition members of the Chamber of Deputies had filed interpellations on the government's handling of the epidemic. The Egyptian Parliament had two houses, the Senate and the Chamber of Deputies. The Wafd dominated both houses, but the opposition had enough representation to put the government on the spot. It normally heard the interpellations, answered them by explaining and defending its policy, and then sought a vote of confidence. This time Nahhas broke with customary procedure and spoke first.

It was an evening session. Mustafa Nahhas marched in, removed his overcoat, gloves, and tarboosh, and began to speak.[27] He led off by claiming that the mosquito had been brought in by increased air or land transport from Sudan because the Mediterranean routes were closed owing to the war. He thus implicated the British in the epidemic. The Ministry of Health had formed two sections, one for treatment, the other for control. The treatment section had fifty doctors, eighty medical assistants, one thousand laboratory assistants, and two thousand other workers. The control section had been organized according to the methods advised by an American doctor who had worked on malaria control in Brazil. Under military orders of January 1943, the government had drained or filled one-fifth of the marshes, rice plantations, and borrow pits along the sides of train tracks and had given out Atabrine, foodstuffs, and, on Faruq's birthday, shoes.[28]

Nahhas repeated that in two years there had been 143,532 cases of malaria in Qina and Aswan, affecting 15 percent of the population, which, he said, numbered 1,115,200. In Qina the death rate had risen from 17.2 per thousand in 1941 to 20.6 per thousand in 1943. In Aswan the death rate had risen from 24.3 per thousand in 1941 to 34.1 per thousand in 1942 to 43.9 per thousand in 1943. This meant an increase of 3,791 deaths over the normal number. Government efforts had, he said, paid off because the epidemic in 1943 was much smaller than in 1942.[29]

Nahhas announced that the Ministry of Social Affairs was planning to open twelve soup kitchens in addition to the existing six to feed 22,400 people. The government would require large factories to feed their workers and to raise wages. He assured the chamber that malaria was not like cholera; it was easy to treat if medication was available and if the people were not malnourished or in need of clothing.[30] He put the blame on the previous government, which had put obstacles in the way of the Wafd's plans to raise the Aswan Dam, to built electricity generators, to strengthen the Isna and Nag'a Hammadi barrages, and to irrigate new land. He said these projects would have eliminated the poverty of Upper Egypt. The large landowners were, he said, responsible for the epidemic because they paid their workers low wages and treated them like slave labor. The Wafd government had decided to distribute land reclaimed in the future to landless fellahin and to raise the minimum daily wage of workers in Qina and Aswan provinces from five to ten piasters.[31]

The government was happy, Nahhas said, to thank the benevolent societies for their missions and Jemima Abbud for her food-distribution project in Armant. The government had supplied the Mabarra and Red Crescent women with rest houses, physicians, transportation, food, and every other assistance required by "such respected ladies who volunteered through humanitarian sentiments though their services were limited."[32] He said the volunteer women worked under the guidance of and in consultation with the government. Furthermore, the Ministry of Waqfs had given one thousand pounds to the Red Crescent and the same amount to the Mabarra Muhammad Ali in 1944. In 1943 the Ministry of Social Affairs had given £E 14,000 to the Red Crescent. In 1944 it gave one thousand pounds to the Mabarra Muhammad Ali, ten thousand to the Red Crescent, and an additional two thousand to the Women's Committee of the Red Crescent. He concluded that the government wanted to recognize those who should be recognized but at the same time wanted to state the facts.[33] Nahhas had spoken for four and one-half hours.

The following night, on 29 February, the opposition had its chance to question the government. Muhammad Sha'rawi, a member of the Sa'dist party, had submitted the first interpellation questioning the condition of public health in the country and its means of improvement.[34] Zuhayr Sabri, Independent Socialist party member and former Wafdist, had submitted the second interpellation questioning the responsibility of the government for the famine and malaria epidemic.[35]

Sha'rawi said that the epidemic had been going on for two years. The government had concealed it until being forced to concede the epidemic's existence following the publicity that surrounded the women's missions and the king's visit. He said that British and American experts had warned the Wafd government of the impending disaster in 1942 and had not accepted their offers of assistance. In addition, he said, Nahhas's statistics were not credible. Mortality was far higher than he had indicated. In the four villages around Luxor, the Mabarra Muhammad Ali women who were working there had reported 809 deaths out of 4,000 inhabitants. Furthermore, even if the number of cases that Nahhas had suggested was correct, the fifty physicians mentioned by Nahhas were not enough. The government should have begun industries and public-works projects to employ the unemployed. It should study the matter of limiting landownership. The epidemic tax, he said, should be on all of the landowners of Egypt not only on those of Upper Egypt because that imbalance implied that the epidemic was a local problem. He then accused the Wafd government of forcing people to donate money for the victims of malaria. He concluded his presentation by reading the article in *al-Ahram* dated 20 December 1943 in which the ministry had announced "success for the gambiae hunters."[36]

Many of the Wafd deputies left while he was speaking, and the Chamber of Deputies was half empty when "sprightly socialist Zuhayr Sabri tripped up to the microphone and brought animation to the debate."[37] He said that the government was not asked to do more than it could, but it should admit when it could not cope. The Wafd projects regarding land development that Nahhas had mentioned had benefited only the landowners. The government claimed it had distributed one million *ukka*s of flour in November and December 1943 in the two provinces that had one million poor people. He said that he had obtained the figure of one million by subtracting the number of taxpayers and their dependents from the total population. That, he pointed out, would make one loaf of bread per year per person.

The minister of supplies interrupted him saying that enough flour for two million loaves had been sent. Sabri replied that that made two loaves of bread per year. Furthermore, he continued, the government's interest in the epidemic really began in January and February 1944, when large quantities of food and clothing were distributed. The people were naked and starving for two years before then. The real problem was hunger, improper distribution of wealth, and projects that destroyed the land of the poor people. He said he had never seen anything like it in the Soviet Union.

After Sabri had concluded, the government had a chance to reply. Fuad Sirag al-Din denied that news of the epidemic had not been known until the women began their work. The Mabarra, he recalled, had left on 19 January 1944, the Red Crescent on 22 January 1944, while *al-Ahram* had mentioned visits by the ministers to the provinces in 1942 and 1943. His government had allowed the press to write and criticize more than it should have, but the opposition had not taken up the call until February. Poverty in the region was not born of the Wafd government; it had been there during the Sirri government too. Furthermore, he pointed out, the Wafd government had on 6 January 1944, which was *before* the women departed, submitted a plan to Parliament for the "epidemic tax" on the wealthy in Upper Egypt. Finally, he announced that the Wafd government would distribute free food for several months or even a year if necessary.[38]

Marcel Colombe, a French historian of modern Egypt, reports that during the debate one of the deputies stated that Egypt was living through terrible hours, that Egypt was being broken on a foreign vise, and that malaria had come to Egypt via British airplanes, while the Wafd government had come via British tanks. This charge was stricken from the parliamentary record, but, Colombe says, it circulated from mouth to mouth, spread by public rumor.[39]

In the end, the Wafd-dominated chamber voted to uphold the actions of the Wafd government, and the interpellation was concluded. The crisis, however, had not ended. The opposition and the king had scored many points, and the government had slipped badly.

The opposition immediately claimed that Nahhas's lengthy defense did not stand up to close scrutiny. The Wafd government, it pointed out, had not directly mentioned malaria in its press announcements about ministers visiting Upper Egypt, and most of the control measures Nahhas had mentioned had been undertaken immediately before the debate.

Meanwhile, Killearn received more reports of deplorable conditions in Upper Egypt. He wrote in his diary that the government had really "bought it this time" and that its negligence seemed "almost criminal."[40] Killearn was clearly worried about his support for the Wafd government backfiring.

Shortly after the debate, Nahhas accused Killearn of letting him down, even though he had made every effort to meet British demands in supporting the war effort. He had furnished food for British troops, he had interned undesirables, only to find himself publicly accused of doing everything the British wanted. Killearn, he said, had put all the blame on the Wafd government in his two communiqués, indicating that British support for the Nahhas government was weakening. Killearn assured him that his policy toward any Egyptian government was based on supporting whoever could provide maximum tranquillity. The British government, he said, did not usually mind taking the blame for the problems of the Egyptian government if it believed that the government was doing its best to solve those problems, but he did not think the government was doing its best to solve the malaria crisis in Upper Egypt.[41] Yet the only alternative to the Wafd government, Killearn reasoned, was a palace regime. The time was therefore not yet ripe to drop the Wafd. It would come when victory in the war was closer at hand or when the Wafd had undermined its position to the extent that the British war effort was hindered.[42] The Wafd government remained in power. It had gained time and now tried to deal with the malaria crisis.

During the Chamber of Deputies debate, Nahhas had issued the military order raising the minimum daily wage of workers in Qina and Aswan provinces from five to ten piasters. Firms employing more than fifty people were required to serve a noontime meal to all workers that was not to cost more than three piasters, half paid by the worker, half by the firm. Under the new policy foodstuffs could not be transferred from one province to another for sale, nor could supplies that were distributed to the poor be sold.[43] A British embassy report on malaria control commented that the military order raising the minimum wage from five to ten piasters daily would not solve the problem because the fellahin were still left at a subsistence level and remained prey to epidemics that a healthy person could easily withstand. The embassy report implicated the entire latifundia system in Upper Egypt by observing that in Upper Egypt half a dozen families owned estates of thousands of feddans, which were worked by fellahin who were paid a minimum wage and had no share in the products of their labor. Food and clothing were rationed and sold at subsidized prices, but the venality of local officials rendered the program useless. There was no remedy, concluded the report, other than a complete social revolution because the Wafd government was unlikely to undertake the necessary reform projects.[44]

The Wafd government, however, did take steps to improve rural public health conditions. Fuad Sirag al-Din announced that social centers were to be established in twenty-five villages, and smaller, locally run service centers—to provide information about proper hygiene, community organization, and education—were to be established in other villages. The Wafd government, he went on to say, was designing model villages that would avoid the unsanitary conditions of the traditional villages and was planning to increase the number of small landowners to help create a middle class that could be a stable and productive force in Egyptian society.[45]

Again rivaling the British and the Wafd in the three-way competition, the palace portrayed itself as the leading force in reforming social and public health conditions in Upper Egypt. Mustafa Amin, the editor of *Ithnayn wa Dunya,* who had accompanied the king on his birthday visit to Upper Egypt, wrote that the week of the parliamentary debate

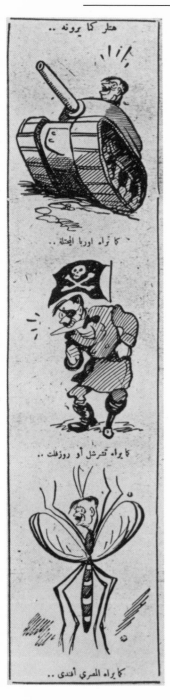

should be called "malaria week" because all the world had felt the mosquito's sting.[46] Although no one in Cairo had been afflicted with the calamity, he said, the parliamentary discussion, the press, and the government declarations had forced everyone to face the problem of poverty. The mosquito's "blessed sting" stimulated the drive to raise the standard of living. Egypt's war against the malaria mosquito was like the war against Hitler and Mussolini (fig. 5). Egypt must mobilize for development, rebuild rural villages, create new rural health centers, and redistribute wealth. Companies that made millions in profits should be required to provide housing, food, and medicine for their workers. The government should impose an inheritance tax, raise the minimum wage, and resume the Aswan Dam electrification project.[47] The point, Mustafa Amin continued, was not to ask who was to blame: everyone wanted to blame some enemy. Egypt needed a "social coup d'état."[48] Foreign farmers lived in ventilated houses, whereas the fellahin's houses were like cemeteries where life and death lived side by side. Egypt was unjust in asking the fellahin to go to school, to get medical care, or even to wear shoes when all were beyond their means. Egypt was unjust in expecting the fellahin to participate in the struggle for nationalism while they were immobilized by poverty, misery, and hardship. In the preceding twenty years, those who had spoken about doing something for the fellahin had really meant doing something for the landowners. Landowners had demanded an increase in the price of cotton and wheat. When prices increased, the owners got richer and the fellahin sank deeper into

Fig. 5. "Hitler as they saw him" as seen (reading top to bottom) by Occupied Europe, as seen by Churchill or Roosevelt, and as seen by Masri Effendi. Source: *Ruz al-Yusuf,* 30 March 1944.

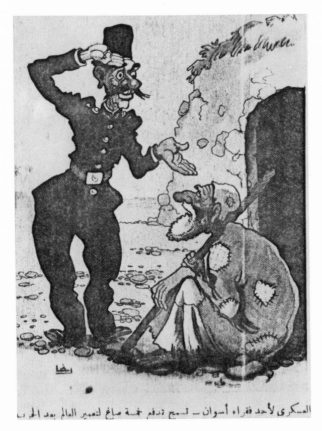

الـمـسـكـرى لأحد فـقـراء أسـوان ــ تـسـمـح تـدفـم خـسـة صاغ لتـعـمـيـر العالم بعد الحرب

Fig. 6. Policeman says to one of the poor in Aswan: "Can you give me 5 piasters to rebuild the world after the war?" Source: *Ithnayn wa Dunya*, 28 February 1944.

poverty.[49] This call to action expressed sentiments that were to intensify in the postwar era (figs. 6–10).

Ruz al-Yusuf published an article entitled "The King and the Fellah," in which the assistant overseer of the royal domain described improvements that had recently been made at the royal estate at Inshas.[50] The fellahin had been given fired (rather than mud) bricks to build their houses and had sanitary facilities and potable water. The land was irrigated by machine. The fellahin shared the crops with the landlord at the unusually favorable rate of 60 percent for the fellah, 40 percent for the owner. The royal estates had hospitals, social services, physicians,

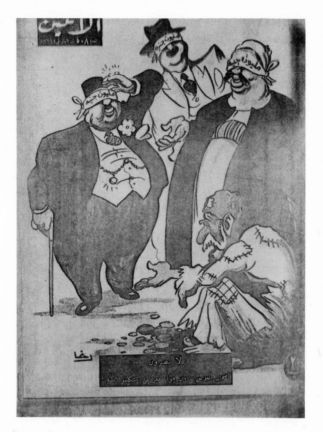

Fig. 7. Reading right to left, a lower-class war profiteer, a foreign entrepreneur, and an *effendi* (member of the wealthy elite), wear blindfolds and do not see the poverty around them. Each blindfold says "A Million Pounds." Source: Cover, *Ithnayn wa Dunya,* 7 March 1944.

and nurses. Workers on the royal estates in Qina and Aswan were paid more than the minimum wage.[51] These improvements were, however, limited to a few model farms, and these were the ones to which visitors were taken.

In response to the malaria epidemic, Mirit Butrus Ghali wrote a series of influential essays about how to combat poverty. He stated that experts should study Egypt's resources and the needs of the people. Then the government should reclaim land; begin industrial projects;

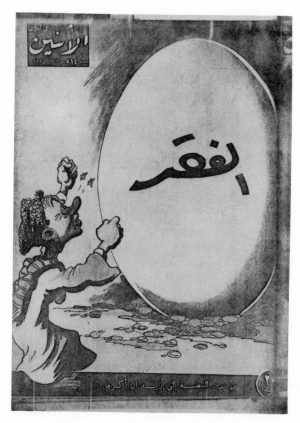

Fig. 8. Ibn al-balad shaking fist at egg called "Poverty": "This is the egg I want to crack."
Source: Cover, *Ithnayn wa Dunya*, 17 April 1944.

upgrade nutrition, housing, clothing, social services, and education; and improve working conditions.[52] In 1945 he published the essays in a study entitled *Agrarian Reform* in which he emphasized that World War II had brought shortages and disastrous epidemics, which had exacerbated the already impoverished conditions in which the rural citizen lived.[53]

Throughout the crisis, *Ithnayn wa Dunya* and *Ruz al-Yusuf* satirized the disparities in Egypt. The editorials and cartoons in the propalace journals often expressed radical ideas for social reform, criticized the wealthy ruling elite, called for justice for the fellahin, for raising the

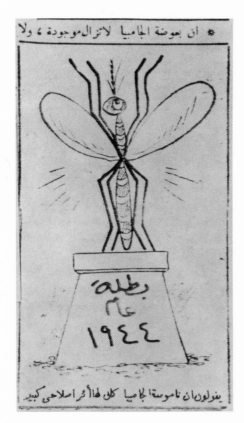

Fig. 9. "Gambiae larvae continue to be found so the malaria mosquito will continue to mobilize great reforms." The malaria mosquito is named "heroine of 1944." Source: *Ruz al-Yusuf*, 20 April 1944.

Fig. 10. Ibn al-balad points to an airplane hangar named "poverty" from which airplanes emerge. Reading right to left they are named "ignorance," "disease," and "weakness." Ibn al-balad comments: "That is the real hangar." Source: *Ithnayn wa Dunya*, 10 July 1944.

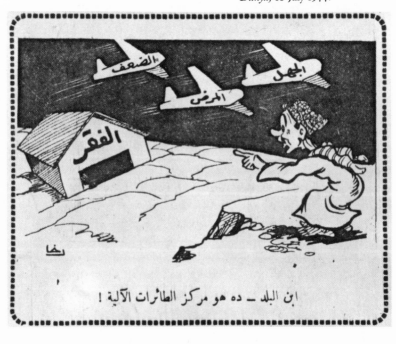

standard of living, and for expanding public health services. The reformist stance of the propalace journals must be seen as an attempt to upstage the Wafd, which claimed to be the party of the people and consistently championed the rights of the disadvantaged.

Following Faruq's birthday trip to Upper Egypt, the palace had come to see itself as a leading advocate of public health reform. It viewed public health reform as a safe cause in which it excelled at the expense of the British, who had a weak record in public health management, and of the Wafdists, who had a weak record in malaria control.

Meanwhile, the Ministry of Health had hastily hired more malaria-control workers, bringing their number to four thousand by the middle of March. It established centers in the larger towns where families could go to register for malaria relief. The Egyptian army detailed thirty men for field eradication work in Adisat ('Udaysat) and al-Dayr. By June, 1,391 officers and men were on duty, filling in *birka*s and disinfecting standing water with Malariol and Paris green and disinfecting means of transport with pyrethrum.[54]

Final arrangements were also made between British medical officers and the Egyptian Ministry of Health to dispatch two British malaria-control units to Upper Egypt. The publicity section of the British embassy made sure that suitable press converage was given to the units.[55]

Politicians rushed to demonstrate their concern for the victims of malaria. The day after the parliamentary debate on malaria, leading members of the opposition Kutla party departed for Luxor, Aswan, and Qina.[56] They visited the Mabarra Muhammad Ali and Red Crescent food-distribution centers, where they gave speeches and posed for pictures. The Kutla party had been collecting funds and supplies for relief of the victims of malaria and now distributed them with much fanfare.

Two weeks later, Nahhas himself set off to visit Upper Egypt. He took along the ministers of justice, public works, education, interior, health, and *waqf*s. After a tumultuous send-off at the Cairo train station, the party traveled to Minya, Manfalut, and Asiut, towns just outside the malaria-infected region. At each station, huge crowds greeted the train. Nahhas and his party were regaled with receptions and parades. Everywhere the ministers distributed sacks of flour, lentils, and beans, as well as clothing and blankets. Nahhas tasted the food being distributed at one of the soup kitchens and ordered a dish of it served to him at a banquet in his honor. He said that the food and clothing distribution would continue through the summer and fall.[57] Back in Cairo crowds who were waiting to greet Nahhas jammed the station. To all appearances it was an enormously successful trip.

The opposition was furious. The National Front, an opposition coalition led by Makram Ebeid, head of the Kutla party; Ahmad Mahir, head of the Sa'dist party; Muhammad Hussayn Haykal, head of the Liberal Constitutionalist party; and Muhammad Hafiz Ramadan, head of the National party, issued its "Appeal Number 2," a polemical condemnation of the Nahhas government.[58] Among other charges, the appeal said that the government had failed to control malaria in Upper Egypt, that medicine and food sent to the victims were being stolen, and that thousands of Egyptians had been allowed to perish.[59] The appeal said that Nahhas and his associates were afraid the British would not support them after the interpellations in Parliament, so they hired Cairo mercenaries to cheer the party as it left the train station. Then they bribed avaricious provincial officials throughout the region to enlarge the staged receptions. Local officials had received written orders to decorate houses and shops with colored lights. People demonstrating for wages had lined the streets. Dissident students were arrested and sent back to their villages, where they stayed under police watch until the trip was over. The National Front claimed that Nahhas, who continually spoke of upholding the constitution, was the first Egyptian to give the British a free hand in Egypt and was even then conspiring with the British to reschedule Britain's war debts to Egypt at Egypt's expense. Finally, the appeal noted that Nahhas had not even reached the malaria-stricken region, having visited cities just north of it.[60]

These criticisms, despite their containing more than an element of truth, did not daunt Nahhas who, on the contrary, considered the trip a great success, so much so that he made a second trip, this time right to Aswan and Qina provinces, where malaria had hit hardest. He took along a smaller party of the ministers of the interior, public works, health, and supplies. Their train carried food and clothing to be distributed to the poor along the way. At the Aswan malaria station, Wakil showed Nahhas charts and maps of the malaria-control work and samples of the antimalarial medicine that the British army had captured from the Germans after the battle of al-Alamein and had given to Egypt as a present. Nahhas met Muhyi al-Din Farid, who had discovered that the malaria mosquito bred on Nile plants. Wakil said that Farid's discovery indicated that Egyptian experts were contributing to scientific advancement. Nahhas recorded his satisfaction in the station's log book.[61]

In Aswan, Khalil Abd al-Khaliq, the undersecretary of health for quarantine administration, told Nahhas that it was now "proven" that British military aircraft had imported the malaria mosquito from Senegal.[62] He said that the Egyptian government should claim compensation at a future peace conference following the war because each Egyptian dead from malaria was as much a war victim as any American or Allied soldier killed on the field of battle. Nahhas replied that the question of the epidemic's source had turned the British against the Wafd.[63]

Advance-party workers arranged for the most enthusiastic welcome of the trip to take place in Qina, a Wafdist stronghold. There, the crowds shouted, "Nahhas has come, malaria has gone," and he assured them that undemocratic forces had proven a failure in Egypt and that people responded to the Wafd. He praised the constitution, which limited the powers of the king, and pledged that it was the mission of the Wafd party to uphold it. The Wafd party was democratic, and absolute rulers could not help people solve their problems. On several occasions he said that the crowds that greeted him at every stop showed that the population of the region had not been wiped out by malaria, disproving the claims of his opponents, and that the wealthy landowners had fled Upper Egypt in fear of the epidemic.[64] He concluded his tour by announcing his intention to establish at Aswan and Qina two facilities, to be named Mustafa Nahhas Institution, for children orphaned by malaria. The orphanages would be endowed with £E 100,000 from Wafd-party funds.[65] This plan later caused the Wafd considerable embarrassment, and the orphanages were never built.[66]

Meanwhile, opposition politicians were heatedly criticizing Nahhas's trips and the content of his speeches. In an open letter to *al-Ahram*, four opposition deputies in the National Front replied that the large landowners and their relatives had taken up the struggle against malaria before the Wafd government had taken action.[67] Many critics wondered how the Wafd treasury, which had been bankrupt in 1942 when the party assumed power, could now bestow lavish endowments on orphanages. Many suspected the source to be the donations collected for malaria victims.

Despite the opposition's allegations, Nahhas's receptions were not entirely staged. The Wafd still retained its reputation from the post–World War I era, when it had led the independence movement against the British. Most observers agreed that the Wafd would still win a majority vote against the other political parties in an open election. Faruq was also popular, but he could not establish or carry out policies and had no access to government revenues. He could only dismiss the government, appoint a new one, and call for general elections.[68]

Faruq was outraged by Nahhas's trips, which seemed to him intentionally designed to upstage the palace. He complained that Nahhas had behaved like royalty in a direct affront to the palace, that he had the special anthems played for him that were, under customary protocol, reserved for the king.[69] Nahhas had, he claimed, gone altogether out of bounds.

On 12 April Faruq called Killearn to Abdin Palace and handed him a carefully prepared memorandum. It began by informing Killearn that Faruq had long wanted to dismiss the Wafd government. Now Nahhas had made claims that both malaria and famine were nearly nonexistent in Upper Egypt. This contention was tantamount to calling the king a liar. The two British communiqués, which had blamed the Wafd government for negligent distribution of food and supplies in Upper Egypt, were entirely correct. The government had spent its funds on propaganda for the Wafd party, for intrigues in al-Azhar University, and for purchase of influence from public officials. Such actions could affect the tranquillity that Faruq knew Killearn needed during wartime. Therefore, the memorandum asked for a change of government. It promised that Faruq would appoint new ministers known for their competence and honesty: none would be a member of a political party. The new government would continue to support the British war effort and after a few months would resign and hold free elections.[70]

Killearn stalled for time by saying that the memorandum had to be officially considered before it could be acted upon. Then he wired Winston Churchill for advice and took a vacation trip to Alexandria. Faruq waited a few days and, not having heard from Killearn, officially signed the rescript dismissing Nahhas on 18 April 1944. The new prime minister was to be Ahmad Hasanayn, chief of the royal cabinet. Mirit Butrus Ghali was to be minister for commerce and industry, and Ali Tawfiq Shusha, permanent undersecretary of health, was nominated to be the minister of health, but he refused the offer because of other obligations.[71]

Faruq was in for a disappointment. Churchill sent word from London that Nahhas should stay in office for a while longer: "His Majesty's Government would almost certainly range themselves against whoever strikes first. Considering that Egypt has, through our exertions, been spared the horrors of invasion and of becoming a battlefield and remains an unravaged peaceful and prosperous land, we have a right to address you on this subject."[72] Upon his return to Cairo, Killearn informed Faruq of this decision and promptly ordered all British commanders in chief to take the necessary steps to make sure their forces were mobilized and ready to give support should the ambassador require it.[73] Faruq rescinded his order dismissing the government, and the crisis was over. The malaria crisis had nearly toppled the government, but British support still held; the Wafd remained in power, and the king had to wait for another day.

This political crisis, however, culminated in the much-discussed invitation to the Rockefeller Foundation. During Faruq's attempt to dismiss the government, Muhammad Hussayn Haykal, leader of the Liberal Constitutionalist party, and three other prominent opposition senators had submitted interpellations in the Senate.[74] After repeating the allegations of negligence made during the earlier debate in the Chamber of Deputies, Haykal brought up a new matter. He said that Dr. Fred Soper, the malaria expert who successfully eradicated malaria in Brazil in the 1930s, had offered his assistance to the Egyptian government in 1943, but the government had refused it. Soper, he said, had recommended a special administration for mosquito eradication within the Ministry of Health. It would enjoy full authority, special wage rates, proper job classifications, and an open budget under an emergency account. Haykal said that the government had only reluctantly accepted help from the British military because of fear of British interference in local affairs. But, he asked, why fear American medical authorities? Senator Mustafa Shurbagi replied that they would also interfere in Egypt's internal affairs.[75] Haykal replied that he did not think interference was the goal of the American medical authorities. The Ministry of Health said the cause of the epidemic was poverty and must be eliminated, but the mosquito, he insisted, must be eradicated as well.[76]

In his reply to the Senate, Nahhas said that collaboration with foreign scientists had never been refused so long as they did not deprive Egyptian experts of responsibility. Dr. Soper's survey had been much appreciated. Foreign doctors were not familiar with the customs and traditions of Egyptian people. Would foreign doctors have exceeded the efforts of Egyptian doctors during the past two years? In any case, Nahhas said, the Ministry of Health had just asked Dr. Soper to return to Egypt to make another survey.[77] This casually delivered statement meant that the Wafd had capitulated at last. The Rockefeller Foundation would be invited to lead the eradication campaign. In the public health sphere, the Americans were to disrupt the three-way power struggle between the British, the Wafd, and the palace.

The politics of malaria had ironically benefited the victims of malaria and famine in Upper Egypt. The government was now allocating vast resources to the antimalaria campaign. For a time, ample food, clothing, blankets, and medications were available free or at reduced cost. Some observed that life was better in emergencies. Perhaps the solution was to find a way to keep public health in the national consciousness. But first malaria had to be conquered.

5

Enter the Rockefeller Foundation

Fred L. Soper, the Rockefeller Foundation expert who had tried to obtain an invitation from the Ministry of Health to lead an eradication program in 1943, believed that a successful program would not only save the lives of countless Egyptians and Allied troops but would also win goodwill for the foundation and for the United States. On the basis of the Brazilian eradication campaign, Soper was already convinced that he could see the program through to success in Egypt. He had, however, encountered formidable political obstacles when he first suggested his plan early in 1943. The severity of the 1943 epidemic had now removed those obstacles, and the Americans moved rapidly in Egypt, as elsewhere, to take advantage of the unusual opportunity. It was an early manifestation of the worldwide American ascendancy that is commonly associated with the postwar era.

A complex exercise in medical politics began on 24 February 1944, when Soper, then stationed in Italy with the U.S.A. Typhus Commission, was reading his copy of *Stars and Stripes,* the U.S. Army newspaper. His eye fell on an article stating that deaths from malaria in Upper Egypt had reached an "extremely high" number.[1] Soper realized that his dire predictions had come true and decided to try again for an invitation to direct a malaria-control project. It would be another feather in his cap after his success in Brazil and would enhance the reputation of the Rockefeller Foundation in Egypt. He let Alexander Kirk, the U.S. minister in Cairo, know that the Rockefeller offer was still good.[2] Four days later, the marathon Chamber of Deputies debate over malaria control precipitated an avalanche of political controversy. To avoid offending either the Wafd or the British embassy, Kirk decided to wait until things settled down before renewing Soper's offer to the Ministry of Health.

Meanwhile the British embassy and the British military authorities were coming around to the point of view that outside assistance was needed in dealing with the malaria epidemic. At the end of March 1944 a British military report stated that, while malaria had indeed hit the malnourished more severely than the healthy, it was nevertheless debilitating and dangerous to everyone. The main effort, the military report said, should be directed toward control, and if possible, toward eradication of the malaria mosquito.[3] Kirk decided the time was right and informed both the British embassy and the Ministry of Health of Soper's new offer.

Killearn had, in fact, come to the conclusion that he needed the Rockefeller Foundation for the same reason that he needed the Wafd party: the war effort. Hundreds of thousands of British troops were in Egypt. A severe malaria epidemic in the Delta could be at least as dangerous to the war effort as a pro-Axis Egyptian government. Killearn had been forced to realize that the British could not offer the necessary expertise at the time and that Soper was probably the world's most experienced malaria eradication expert. These facts overrode his fears of American encroachment in Egypt, at least for the moment. Therefore, Killearn had informed Amin Osman, the Wafdist minister of finance and liaison to the British embassy, that the Wafd government must extend the invitation to the Rockefeller Foundation. Killearn warned Osman that if the government did not accept the Rockefeller Foundation's offer public opinion would turn against it.[4] This conversation took place the day Faruq informed Killearn that he had decided to dismiss the Wafd government. Nahhas was in no position to resist British pressure.

Faruq himself had decided the government should extend the invitation to the Rockefeller Foundation. For weeks, women from the Mabarra Muhammad Ali had been pressuring the palace on behalf of the foundation because Chevikar, at the first news of the epidemic, had contacted Claude Barlow, a well-known Rockefeller Foundation bilharzia expert who had worked in Egypt for many years. She asked him to recommend an Egyptian malaria expert to her. Barlow introduced Muhyi al-Din Farid—who before the war had worked in malaria control with the Rockefeller Foundation—to Chevikar and her husband, Ilhami Husayn Pasha. Farid in turn informed her that "only Soper" could do the job of malaria control. Chevikar and the volunteers accordingly urged Faruq to pressure Wakil to recruit him.[5] For his part, the king may have believed that the American foundation would upstage both Wafdist and British efforts in malaria control. The malaria epidemic had become one of his best weapons against the Wafd.

On 11 April, the day before Faruq tried to dismiss the Wafd government, Kirk had reported to Washington, D.C., that the official invitation was "still hanging fire."[6] He said that the king and other influential people were pressuring the government to extend the invitation to the Rockefeller Foundation. Wakil, he thought, was in no mood to accept help from the British, but the king was recommending the Rockefeller Foundation as a neutral organization. Kirk raged that "the bugbear of foreign penetration" was keeping the government from extending the invitation, thereby endangering the health of the entire nation.[7] The Egyptians had, however, suffered from foreign domination for many years and were more than a little suspicious of further high-power participation in their internal affairs.

The pressure from the palace and from the British embassy finally forced Wakil to capitulate. He contacted Kirk and worked out an agreement.[8] On 13 April, the day after Faruq's attempted dismissal, the Rockefeller Foundation through the U.S. State Department received an invitation to participate in a conference on malaria control.[9] The conference would be followed by a firm invitation to the Rockefeller Foundation. Soper made preparations to return to Egypt from Italy.

Killearn then informed Eden that he had supported the Rockefeller proposal because the foundation was well qualified for such work and because it would have been difficult to refuse on political grounds.[10] He said he had always supported the idea of including Americans along with British experts in fieldwork in Upper Egypt so that American critics would not be able to say that they would have been able to do better had they not been prevented from participating.[11] He cautioned that the British should not appear to be avoiding the assistance of the Rockefeller Foundation, which was internationally known for its work in malaria control.[12] He then tried to forestall further American involvement (as will be seen below). He was trying to walk a tightrope: he wanted to defeat malaria *and* keep the Americans out of Egypt. Thus, he needed the Americans for the moment, but he feared their long-term presence. This dilemma was an example of the British predicament in the Middle East during and after World War II.

Nahhas made one last try to back out of the invitation. He sent word through Amin Osman to Killearn that he thought it best not to encourage Egyptian ministries to deal with the Americans, who often approached the Ministries of Health and Agriculture with offers of assistance. Killearn replied that, given the reputation of the Rockefeller Foundation, the public would have reacted very negatively if the government had refused its assistance.[13]

Early in May Wakil telephoned Farid at his home in Helwan to tell him he was sending a car for him. When the two were together, the minister told Farid that the government was in a jam. On the one hand, he said, the king wanted to get rid of the Wafd government. On the other hand, the Americans wanted to step in with a new imperialism and to colonize Egypt. Now Soper was coming again to investigate the malaria epidemic. Wakil said that Farid had been his student in medical school and had also worked before with the Rockefeller Foundation. He wanted Farid to accompany Soper on his trip up the Nile and show him what the ministry had done but to avoid places that were badly infested with *A. gambiae*, such as the region from Isna south. Farid and Soper would find a well-equipped boat waiting at Nag'a Hammadi. Wakil asked him to sail upriver in the center to avoid the infested areas. It was essential, he said, that Soper write a report favorable to the Ministry of Health. Farid replied that he would try but that it would not be easy given the situation in the malaria-stricken region.[14]

Wakil then gave Farid a written memo with three points: Soper should be asked to be careful in phrasing his report to avoid having political capital made of it should it become public; any doctors doing good work should be mentioned; and Soper should know that, were he to consent to becoming a consultant of the Ministry of Health, he could have any salary he desired.[15] In this way Wakil hoped that the report would be positive in tone.

On 7 May Soper arrived back in Egypt. There, Soper learned that

Faruq had sent word to the U.S. legation that he wanted Soper presented at court.[16] At the audience at Abdin Palace, Faruq told him that the catastrophic proportions of the epidemic had made malaria a question of political importance of great concern to him and that a royal commission had visited the infected zones and calculated that in two years there had been one hundred thirty thousand malaria deaths. The king assured him that "interest, finances, and authority would not be lacking for the attack on the invader."[17]

Soper then set off for Upper Egypt, accompanied by Farid and two assistants. In Aswan Soper found that control work was ongoing but poorly organized. An Egyptian army antimalaria unit was working at Adisat, across the river from Armant. A British army antimalaria unit was stationed at the sugar estate of Abbud Pasha and had been operating there for three weeks. Another British unit (for surveying only) was at the time in Asiut, and a third British unit worked in Cairo as an independent check on the other units. To the embarrassment of the British unit, Farid found gambiae breeding at a distance of only five minutes' walk from its headquarters at Armant.[18]

When Soper and his party returned to Cairo after completing the survey, Wakil contacted Farid to see how the trip had gone. Farid told him that Soper had insisted on going about on his own, checking here and there, and had learned the true extent of the malaria. Wakil was alarmed. But Farid assured him that he had told Soper that politics were involved and that if he criticized the ministry it would impede the whole gambiae-control program. Soper had promised Farid that he would give one copy of his report to the Ministry of Health and keep the other copy himself. He would not submit a report directly to the palace. The ministry could then edit the report and send it on to the king. Wakil was greatly relieved.[19]

In his report Soper said that gambiae was spread over a region at least as large as in 1943. Another equally or more devastating epidemic could be expected in the fall of 1944 and in subsequent years in a wider area, including Lower Egypt, if the gambiae mosquito was not eradicated. The project was entirely feasible: only good administration was necessary. He outlined weaknesses in eradication procedures, made recommendations for reorganization, and listed his conditions for taking over administration of the gambiae eradication program. He insisted on being able to hire, fire, and promote workers to avoid the inefficiency and favoritism that he felt had weakened the service. The ministry should make available transportation and necessary materials. The Rockefeller Foundation would work under the direction of the Ministry of Health but would insist on complete autonomy in running the anti-gambiae campaign. The treatment service would remain the responsibility of the Ministry of Health.[20]

In turn, the Ministry of Health asked the Rockefeller Foundation to avoid publicizing its nearly independent administrative responsibility in organizing and directing the gambiae eradication service. Wakil wanted to avoid negative publicity by keeping the Rockefeller role out of the press while quieting the government's critics for the failure to control the epidemic. The ministry insisted on paying for the entire gambiae eradication service. It allocated £E 200,000, later to be increased to £E 500,000, for the project. Wakil hoped to avoid excessive foreign control by funding the project and by keeping it under the auspices of the Ministry of Health. The Rockefeller Foundation would pay only the salaries of the staff it sent. On 28 May 1944 the terms for collaboration between the Rockefeller Foundation and the Ministry of Health were formally agreed upon.[21]

Meanwhile the British Ministry of Health circulated a file about malaria in Egypt among medical officials in London, seeking opinions on what to do about the epidemic. The British medical officer of health, Port of London, asked whether the recommendations that had been made in March 1944 by the military medical corps had been implemented, and if so, would not the Rockefeller Foundation merely duplicate work already being done? The officer believed the British army in Egypt could offer malaria experts, trained workers, and supplies, while the Rockefeller Foundation had been working in Egypt for many years without much improvement in the Egyptian public health service. He thought the British should use the malaria epidemic as an opportunity to train and closely supervise the Egyptian field staff. Why invite the Rockefeller Foundation in to do much the same thing?[22] In fact, the three British malaria units were limited in size and competence and were able to survey only a very small portion of the malaria-infected region. The British military did not have the experience and resources to compete with the Rockefeller Foundation. The invitation went forward.

Killearn, despite his initial opposition to the Rockefeller Foundation, took all the credit for this outcome. In his diary, he wrote, "The Egyptians with their absurdities of national *amour-propre* were definitely opposed at first to accepting the Rockefeller offer, and I am fairly certain that if I had not taken a very strong line with them, they would eventually have turned it down. As I pointed out in the strongest terms at the time, this would have placed them in a quite impossible position not only vis-à-vis their own people but in the eyes of the whole civilized world. It is satisfactory that this strong medicine should have worked."[23] This statement, referring to the Wafd government's intransigence, was clearly written for public consumption. He presumably hoped not to be held accountable in any way for the public health crisis.

Wakil then held a press conference to discuss the malaria epidemic. He said the poor in Qina and Aswan provinces were better fed and clothed than they had been in the previous year and were thus more capable of tolerating attacks of malaria. The Rockefeller Foundation was, he said, loaning a technical expert whose salary and expenses it would pay. Soper, he said, had again surveyed Upper Egypt and had recorded a distinct improvement over what he had seen during his two surveys in January and April 1943. The epidemic, Wakil said, had been very severe, especially among the poor farm workers on the large sugarcane estates. The government, he added, had saved thousands of lives through its distribution of free food, clothing, and medicine and would continue the distribution the following malaria season.[24]

Wakil had tried to present the malaria situation in a favorable light. He stressed the Ministry of Health's great efforts in dealing with the epidemic and said conditions had improved. The previous month he had announced that the government would spend £E 200 million on new model villages, artesian wells, and public-health centers for each fifteen thousand inhabitants, following examples set by agricultural countries, such as Poland, Romania, and Yugoslavia. Projects designed to eliminate bilharzia and hookworm, which affected 75 percent and 50 percent of the rural people, respectively, would receive £E 4 million.[25] While he again followed the Wafd party's line and blamed the large landowners for exploiting the fellahin, he did not call for land reforms, nor did he explain from where the funds for his reforms were to come. He had high hopes and good intentions, but he lacked the necessary resources for such reforms and the practical knowledge of how to deal with malaria.

On 9 July 1944 two Americans, J. Austin Kerr, a Rockefeller Foundation malaria expert, and Stuart S. Stevenson, a young doctor and conscientious objector doing alternate military service, arrived in Cairo and were taken to Shepheard's Hotel. Bruce Wilson, a Canadian malaria expert with the Rockefeller Foundation who had worked with Soper in Brazil, was to join the staff after completing a project in East Africa. Louis A. Riehl, an American entomologist stationed in Italy with the U.S.A. Typhus Commission, was later seconded to Egypt. Soper spent the first few months in Egypt and visited several times during the operation but left local administration to Kerr and Wilson.

With the Rockefeller Foundation in charge, the American and British military authorities, the Middle East Supply Centre, and the Foreign Economic Administration in Cairo proceeded to release scarce chemicals, the insecticide pyrethrum, and vehicles to the Egyptian government. The new insecticide DDT was superior to pyrethrum but was not yet available for civilian use.[26]

On 15 July the ministry issued an order making Kerr head of the Gambiae Eradication Service in Cairo, Wilson director of field operations, and Farid subdirector. The Gambiae Eradication Service was detached from the Gambiae Treatment Service, and the ministry released the promised one-half million pounds to the new Rockefeller-administered Gambiae Eradication Service. In addition, the senate approved £E 675,000 for relief of malaria victims.[27]

S. Pinkney Tuck, the new American minister who had replaced Alexander Kirk in May 1944, reported to Washington, D.C., that malaria had ceased to be a political issue and that his series of reports would cease "barring unexpected flarebacks."[28] And for a few months there were fewer articles in the press and fewer debates in Parliament. The public considered the malaria crisis at an end. Stamp collectors asked the post office to issue a stamp commemorating the battle against malaria, but it was decided that too many special issues would lower Egypt's reputation in the stamp-collecting world.[29]

Soper meanwhile proceeded to seek out influential persons in the Ministry of Health, in other branches of government, in the foreign embassies, and in society. At a dinner party at the home of the American embassy's cultural attaché, an American Red Cross representative told Soper that the Red Crescent and Mabarra Muhammad Ali volunteers had played an active role both in dealing with the epidemic and in securing the invitation. Soper parried by saying that he thought some-one should "write up the experience of the girls during the gambiae episode."[30]

Later at a dinner with the Butrus Ghali family, he met Gertrude Butrus Ghali, who had gone to Isna with the first group of volunteers. She gave Soper a copy of her diary describing conditions in Isna. Soper read it and concluded that the women's missions were significant only because the women saw for the first time what conditions were like among the poor of Upper Egypt.[31] Little did he suspect how crucial the volunteers were to become to the Rockefeller staff. According to Kerr, "the ladies of high families sold the Rockefeller Foundation to Faruq and became their most valued allies."[32]

The volunteer women also maintained excellent relations with the American army. In August 1944, Nahid Sirri, head of the Women's Committee of the Red Crescent, organized a benefit performance by the U.S. Army's all-soldier musical revue, "This Is the Army," written and directed by Irving Berlin. The performance was a gala event at-tended by Faruq, Killearn, and the other leading personalities of Cairo. All proceeds of the evening went to the Mabarra Muhammad Ali and the Red Crescent.[33]

The Rockefeller Foundation also maintained close ties to the U.S. Army, a fact that was emphasized when Kerr decided that the four Rockefeller staff members should wear American army uniforms that the army under special circumstances allowed civilians to wear. The uniforms hid the fact that the four were there as civilians working for a private organization, but Kerr thought that the advantages out-weighed that disadvantage: the uniforms would distinguish them from the British and were comfortable and convenient to wear. That Wilson was Canadian caused a problem, but the army decided that he could wear it. Soper, however, wore civilian clothes because he thought that they helped his work as a Rockefeller Foundation representative in the Mediterranean region.[34]

Soper made every effort to cultivate good relations with Wakil and other officials in the Ministry of Health and in the government, and he instructed his staff to do likewise. At the outset of the campaign, Soper told Wakil that it was too late in the year for complete eradication, that he should expect another epidemic in the fall, but that total eradication should be completed in 1945. By this time, malaria had again been found in Badari, a region that had been cleared earlier in the year.[35] Soper accordingly instructed Kerr to give particular attention to Badari in hopes of eradicating the mosquito, thus avoiding the predicted malaria outbreak in the fall of 1944.

Kerr set off for Badari where to his surprise he found that the ministry was following the manual Soper had left behind in 1943. The manual had been written after the Rockefeller Foundation's campaign in Brazil as a historical document and for use in antimalarial campaigns in sub-Saharan Africa.[36] The Egyptians had translated the Portuguese administrative titles into Arabic and had already organized its work crews according to the manual, making administration much easier for the Rockefeller staff.[37] The crews were, however, still relying on Malariol to eradicate the larvae. Kerr immediately ordered the changeover from Malariol to Paris green. Paris green required fewer workers, so the eradication service released about one thousand of the four thousand workers.[38]

Under the terms of the agreement, the Rockefeller staff could hire and fire Gambiae Eradication Service employees on the basis of competence alone. Workers were well paid, and those who performed well were promoted rapidly. Those who did not were dismissed with no possibility of appeal. This treatment was not customary in Egypt, and there were many complaints and occasional threats of violence.[39] Nevertheless, morale remained high. Eric Pridie, a British embassy medical expert, visited the Asiut headquarters a year later in August 1945 and reported that Bruce Wilson, the field director, was good at handling the staff and that his staff had also learned to handle him to perfection. The result "was a very happy atmosphere."[40] In a longer report prepared a few days later, he reflected that the Rockefeller Foundation staff had succeeded because they rigorously controlled their subordinate workers by an elaborate system of checks and discharged them immediately for neglect of duty or for inefficiency. They also treated the workers as human beings and rewarded competence with promotions and increased salaries. In consequence, he concluded, the Gambiae Eradica-

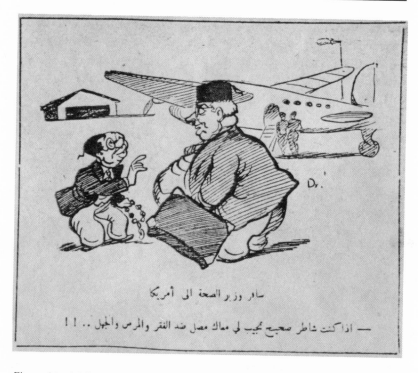

سافر وزير الصحة الى أمريكا

— اذا كنت شاطر صحيح تجيب لي معاك مصل ضد الفقر والمرض والجهل .. ! !

Fig. 11. Masri Effendi to Wakil on his departure to the United States: "Bring us back a vaccine against poverty." Source: *Ruz al-Yusuf,* 30 July 1944.

tion Service workers had a sense of pride in their work.[41] He did not realize that the high salaries commanded by the eradication workers were possible on an emergency basis only because Egypt lacked both the resources and the facilities to sustain such an effort on a long-term basis.

Just after the Rockefeller Foundation had begun work, the U.S. State Department, to cement the new friendship between Wakil and the United States, had sponsored him on a six-week tour of medical facilities in the United States. Such scientific visits were and are a common part of foreign policy. Masri Effendi, the cartoon character depicting the typical urban gentleman, reminded readers of the deeper problem. He asked Wakil to bring back a vaccine against poverty (fig. 11).

Upon his return, Wakil made an official visit to inspect the new

Gambiae Eradication Service field organization. Kerr accompanied him on a special train, which was greeted at every stop with police on parade, bands, and crowds cheering and waving their cards from the Gambiae Treatment Service. Kerr learned that there had been a rumor that, if people presented their cards, they would each receive a free blanket. Wakil visited two relief kitchens at Qurna, part of the Luxor administration. One greatly displeased him, and he promised that the government would improve it. The other, run by the Red Crescent, was managed by a competent woman and was dispensing bread, cheese, oil, dates, and green onions. Wakil found it very satisfactory. Kerr observed that the danger of starvation had long since passed but that for political reasons free food distribution had been continued by the government.[42]

Back in Cairo, Wakil announced that each family in the malaria-stricken region had received a treatment card to ensure accurate statistics, that the ministry had distributed eight million Atabrine tablets, and that they had held another two million in reserve. Schools, he said, had been converted to hospitals where necessary.[43] His efforts to impress the public came to nothing. By early October he was frantically seeking promotions and fellowships for physicians whom he favored.[44] He knew his government was in jeopardy.

In October 1944 with the outcome of the war no longer in doubt, the British embassy withdrew its support for Nahhas and the Wafd government. Faruq had finally gotten his way. While Killearn was conveniently away on vacation, Faruq issued a royal order dismissing the government.[45] A new government was formed by a coalition of minority parties (Sa'dist, Liberal Constitutionalist, Kutla) and independents. It had come to power with the support of the palace. Kerr was anxious to learn the new government's attitude toward the Rockefeller Foundation's presence in Egypt. He immediately went to the Ministry of Health to pay his respects to newly appointed Minister of Health Ibrahim Abd al-Hadi, a lawyer and deputy chief of the Sa'dist party. Abd al-Hadi said he hoped for continued cooperation with the Rockefeller Foundation.[46]

Ahmad Mahir, the new prime minister and chief of the Sa'dist party, was anxious to demonstrate his government's greater concern for public health. He announced plans to spend ten million pounds on health programs, to convert existing health centers into public hospitals, and to build more hostels, clinics, and tuberculosis sanitoriums.[47]

Wakil immediately offered to help the new minister of health.[48] But on 31 October 1944, at the age of fifty, Wakil suddenly died of typhoid. He had made a valiant effort to reform Egypt's rural public health services but was diverted by the malaria epidemic and limited by the political weakness of his government. Later governments put into effect many of his ideas and expanded the programs he had initiated.

Two days after the Wafd government fell, the Asiut station wired the Cairo office to inform them that the northernmost section of the Badari district—a section that had been cleared in September—had gambiae once again. By the end of October an epidemic of malaria in Badari was raging with a thousand new cases reported every day. The Badari district had sixty-one villages and a population of about one hundred thousand. On 14 November *A. gambiae* was reported in and around the town of Aswan, and the eradication service was most discouraged.

By mid-November at least twenty thousand new cases were reported in Badari. Mysteriously, very few deaths were reported. Malaria workers investigated and found that most of the new cases were in fact relapsing fever that had been misdiagnosed as malaria. The rest of the cases in Badari were either relapses of falciparum malaria or a milder, non-malignant form of the disease.[50] Only a few were new cases of falciparum malaria and were ascribed to inefficiency in eradication. The minister of health asked the Mabarra and the Red Crescent to assist again in the distribution of free food and blankets in the stricken region. The Red Crescent set up relief stations in Badari and Armant.[51] The Mabarra continued to work in Asiut, where its officers were adjacent to the eradication service's field headquarters.

By the fall of 1944 the pattern of case reporting had reversed. At the beginning of the epidemic people had been reluctant to report their deaths to the authorities. Now with the distribution of free food, clothing, and most popular of all, blankets, people had learned to exaggerate their illness in the hope of receiving the much-needed goods. It became customary to arrive at the distribution centers in tattered clothes to collect the free supplies and then to sell them on the black market. Kerr informed the New York office that the malaria outbreak in Badari was mired in politics. When he visited the region, he had found little true distress and concluded that because of the impending elections, politicians were exaggerating conditions to secure free food and clothing for their constituents.[52]

Despite Kerr's assurances to the Rockefeller Foundation in New York, there were new cases of falciparum malaria in Badari.[53] Eradication had been less than complete, and the Gambiae Treatment Service sent in a report to the Ministry of Health that the Gambiae Eradication Service was inefficient and extravagant.[54]

Just when help was needed it arrived in the form of Habib Doss, a prominent landowner in Asiut, who invited the Rockefeller staff to dinner. Firdaws Shitta and Amina Sidqi of the Mabarra Muhammad Ali also attended. Kerr described the women as leading feminists. He said they were very emancipated, though Muslims, and very Egyptian. One of them, he observed, took a cocktail, and both smoked. A third activist, Mary Kahil, who Kerr thought took orders from Princess Chevikar, had left for Cairo a few days earlier. Kerr remarked that the women were so influential and secure in their position as members of the privileged class that they were fearless.[55] He told them of the treatment service's report and asked for their help. The Mabarra sent in a report to the Ministry of Health stating that the Gambiae Treatment Service was engaged in corrupt practices, and in consequence the ministry called in its director for an explanation. Unfavorable reports by the treatment service against the eradication service stopped abruptly.[56]

Kerr then asked Farid to arrange a meeting with Princess Chevikar to cement relations. At their meeting, Chevikar told him that she was responsible for the invitation to the Rockefeller Foundation and promised to have Kerr presented at Abdin Palace.[57] Three weeks later, Kerr had his audience with the king. After tripping on the rug five paces in front of Faruq, Kerr managed to salute and was formally introduced. Kerr informed the king that, while gambiae had not yet been eradicated, the danger of another serious epidemic was past. The quantity of Atabrine distributed in Badari, he said, testified to the efficiency of the treatment service rather than to the number of persons ill with malaria. Faruq offered his complete support, and Kerr found him "most charming and friendly."[58] Kerr then let it be known that the meeting had gone well and that the king had assured him of his backing.[59]

Relations between the Rockefeller Foundation, the Ministry of Health, and the volunteers were solidified in January when the Ministry of Health doctors at Luxor hosted an elegant tea at the Winter Hotel for Ali Tawfiq Shusha. Makram Ebeid, the minister of finance, several of the volunteer women, and the Rockefeller staff attended the tea. The women wore the Red Crescent uniform, which Kerr described in his diary. "The cloak is light gray. The hat is a disk-like affair, with gray sides to match the cloak, and a red felt top. Quite natty and distinctive, and yet quite different from anything I have seen the Red Cross ladies wear in other countries."[60] Their professional appearance appealed to him.

Kerr was sometimes struck by the contrast between the standard of living of the elite women and that of the poor majority in Egypt. On 11 February 1945, one year after King Faruq had made his famous birthday visit to the malaria-stricken regions of Upper Egypt, Princess Chevikar held a lavish birthday party for him at her palace in Cairo. After attending the party Kerr wrote in his diary, "the most awe-inspiring natural phenomenon that I have ever seen is the Grand Canyon of the Colorado River. The sociological implications of the lavishness of the party, contrasted with the rampant squalor of Egypt, seem to me to be comparable in degree to the geological implications of the Grand Canyon."[61]

The close association between the elite women and the Rockefeller staff continued. Kerr attended a reception arranged by Jemima Abbud for the Red Crescent at the Anglo-Egyptian Union. There, Kerr met Nahid Sirri and her husband, Husayn Sirri, the former prime minister. He found that Sirri was very proud of his wife's activities and that the general attitude toward the women's work was one of admiration.[62] The volunteer women continued to associate with and to support the Rockefeller staff who ran into no further difficulties.

By the end of the year the Gambiae Eradication Service was on its way to success. It had reorganized the ministry's *darakat* (disinfection zones) and reduced their number from about 900 to 641. It then regularly monitored the *darakat,* checking and rechecking to ensure that each was systematically treated with Paris green. The eradication service kept extensive records, which were continually monitored for accuracy. In September 1944 the Ministry of Health received sixty-eight tons of

Paris green through the Middle East Supply Centre, enabling the eradication service to discontinue its use of Malariol.[63] Teams periodically disinfected railroad cars and automobiles with pyrethrum and with DDT, which had become available for civilian use in November 1944.[64]

The Gambiae Treatment Service, which was run by the Ministry of Health, not by the Rockefeller Foundation, divided the infected region into sixteen treatment zones administrated from Luxor. Teams went house-to-house searching for patients, dispensed drugs "on the spot," and carried out extensive "health propaganda" through films and radio broadcasts to explain how to prevent malaria, to urge people to seek early treatment, and to convince them to continue taking the medication for the correct period of time.[65]

In December 1944 eradication service workers were finding fewer and fewer foci of gambiae larvae. In January 1945 only 37 of the 641 *darakat* were infested with *A. gambiae* larvae. In February only three darakat were infested.[66] The last foci was found on 19 February 1945 by an Egyptian crew working in a remote section near Armant.[67] During the spring and summer, eradication workers continued searching for larvae, spreading Paris green over pools of standing water, checking water samples, and recording results. At the beginning of September 1945 the eradication service stopped all control work to see if the mosquito had reappeared following the summer floods. No foci were found.[68]

In early November 1944 Kerr had predicted that many people would believe that the gambiae mosquito had disappeared because of the cold weather.[69] As predicted, in February 1945 the *Egyptian Gazette* announced that cold temperatures had killed the malaria and that the Ministry of Health was making preparations to control the disease before the next malaria season. Kerr observed that fifteen tons of Paris green per month had also helped put an end to the malaria season.[70]

The minister of health could hardly wait to announce the final eradication of the malaria mosquito. It was quite a coup over the previous ministry. In October he jumped the gun a bit and announced that the malaria mosquito had been completely eradicated from Egyptian territory and that the ministry would take every means to prevent its return.[71] In December, when further checking indicated that no *A. gambiae* had returned with the annual flood, the service was disbanded.

Kerr circulated a letter that told the workers, soon to lose their well-paying jobs, that the eradication service had been like an army mobilized against an invader. Now that the invader had been annihilated, demobilization was inevitable. Muhyi al-Din Farid read the letter to the assembled workers in Asiut and added that the money they had earned was *halal* (legal under Islamic law, as opposed to *haram* or forbidden).[72] About two thousand workers had lost their jobs. Relief work carried out by the Ministry of Supply, the Mabarra Muhammad Ali, and the Red Crescent was terminated.[73]

The Gambiae Eradication Service had spent more than £E 400,000 and had used 137 tons of Paris green. The means of organization and the carefully monitored system of checking and cross-checking had proved successful: the mosquito had been eradicated only seven months after the effort had begun, and measures were being taken to ensure against its reappearance.

On 4 January 1946 Ibrahim Abd al-Hadi hosted a dinner at Groppi's, a famous restaurant in Cairo, to celebrate the eradication of gambiae. Two hundred fifty people attended, including Ali Tawfiq Shusha, the permanent undersecretary of health; Khalil Abd al-Khaliq, the undersecretary of health for quarantine administration; other Ministry of Health officials; and the ministers of supplies, social welfare, and defense. Tuck, Soper, Kerr, and representatives from the British embassy and army attended. Fourteen women from the Mabarra Muhammad Ali and the Red Crescent attended. Princess Aisha represented Chevikar, head of the women's section of the Mabarra, and was seated to the right of the minister of health in the place of honor. Nahid Sirri sat on his left. Amina Sidqi, Sophie Butrus Ghali, and Jemima Abbud were among the guests. The male members of the women's households did not receive invitations—an unusual move for the time—in recognition of the women's independent contribution to the malaria campaign.[74]

Shusha and Kerr gave speeches, which were broadcast on the radio. Shusha said that Egypt had become aware of gambiae's plan of conquest, to sneak in from central Africa and destroy everything, but Egypt had stopped it before it was too late.[75] Kerr described the organization of the Gambiae Eradication Service. The eradication project had been expensive, he said, but it had cost Egypt far less than would have the losses in human life and crops.[76]

Soon after the celebrations the ministry established its Insect Eradication Section to utilize the well-trained personnel of the Gambiae Eradication Service to carry out other mosquito eradication projects and to study means of fly control.[77] The Ministry of Health also established three malaria stations between Aswan and the border with Sudan, and Egyptian and Sudanese authorities agreed to exchange information about the spread of *A. gambiae* downriver from Sudan.[78]

The victory over malaria was made possible by a fortuitous combination of scientific and administrative expertise, hard work, and political circumstances. It was the first time that malaria eradication workers had been able to stamp out an epidemic that had spread into inhabited terrain, citrus orchards, plantations, and irrigation canals. On the basis of the Egyptian campaign, Soper, ignoring the wider social context, concluded that total eradication of malaria was a technical problem requiring only good administration, adequate funds, and DDT.[79]

Government officials and ministry experts in both the Wafdist and propalace governments, the physicians and other medical personnel, the field workers in the eradication and treatment services, the volunteers of the Mabarra Muhammad Ali and the Red Crescent, and the British army medical corps had all contributed to the victory. The Rockefeller Foundation staff had only directed and brought to completion the final stages of the eradication work. With the exception of the salaries of the Rockefeller staff members, the Egyptian government had paid all of the campaign expenses.

A few months later, King Faruq issued medals to those who had participated in fighting the epidemic: 724 went to individuals in the Ministry of Health; 87 to the Ministry of Public Works; 70 to the Railway Service; 37 to the Ministry of Social Affairs; 33 to the Ministry of Commerce and Industry; 47 to the Red Crescent; 40 to the Mabarra Muhammad Ali; 95 to the British army; and 5 to the Rockefeller staff members.[80] In addition, the queen gave each of the women a small pin encrusted with jewels.[81] The Egyptian army refused to accept any medals because, it insisted, it had only done its duty. No medals went to officials of the former Wafd government.

The eradication campaign had demonstrated the usefulness of private voluntary organizations, both international and domestic, and had again reinforced the political importance of public health. Its success had strengthened the position of the palace; the propalace government; the volunteer women; and, through the success of the Rockefeller Foundation, the Americans. Conversely, it had weakened the positions of the Wafd and the British. The Wafd could only await its chance to return to power. The British embassy now sought to regain its prominence in Egypt's public health sphere.

6

British-American Rivalries

During and after World War II, American political, economic, and military power began to threaten British predominance in the Middle East and elsewhere.[1] For Lord Killearn, an early warning of the new and unwelcome political relationship came in the public-health sphere. He decided to fight back.

In May 1944, while urging the Wafd government to extend the invitation to the Rockefeller Foundation, Killearn had hastily tried to alert the foreign office to the danger of American encroachment in Egypt. With evident resentment, he had written Anthony Eden a letter reminding him that he had predicted in 1943 that, if the British did not take immediate action, "international enterprise might in the future interest itself in the health problems of Egypt."[2] This prediction, he said, had now become a reality and a "galaxy" of American medical and scientific experts had eclipsed British efforts. He informed Eden that a British medical research institute would remove the necessity for further foreign (American) assistance. Furthermore, the institute, being independent of the British government, could give informal advice to the Egyptian government. Killearn enclosed in the letter a report prepared by the British embassy detailing the need for specialized British medical and scientific research facilities in Egypt.

The report said that the war had revealed many inadequacies in medical and scientific research in Egypt with regard to the welfare of both British troops and Egyptian civilians. Realizing they needed assistance, the Egyptians had asked for help from the Royal Army Medical

Corps in dealing with malaria. There were, however, deficiencies in the British facilities, and so the United States of America had "responded to the call as if by accident or design and supplied our deficiencies in skilled personnel and equipment" by the provision of internationally known scientists from the U.S.A. Typhus Commission and the U.S. Army Virus Commission.[3] In addition to General Leon A. Fox, director of the U.S.A. Typhus Commission, and Dr. Fred Soper himself, two internationally known poliomyelitis researchers, John Paul and A. B. Sabin, had worked in Egypt. If Britain were to "continue to command the respect and admiration of the Near Eastern countries outside the political sphere," a research institute and experts were needed.[4] The institute could monitor postwar epidemic diseases. "We should be failing in our obligations and acknowledged superior intellectual position if we did not make adequate provision for dealing with any contingencies that may arise from this quarter in the years to come."[5] The proposed institute would be without political influence or intrigue and would bring business to British pharmaceutical companies. The human and animal pathological materials in Egypt would be of interest to British researchers. Furthermore, Egypt was situated on lines of communication to the Far East, and the research institute could become "an instrument of our future imperial policy in the widest sense of the term" for British prestige and for British postwar planning.[6] As a parting shot, the embassy report warned that two eminent Soviet bacteriologists, Professor Smorodinstef, of the U.S.S.R. Institute of Medical Research, and General Professor Solovief, consulting bacteriologist, Siberian Armies, had just visited Egypt to ascertain the state of medical research.[7] Not only the Americans but also the Soviets were sending high-level scientific personnel to Egypt. It was a sign of the new bigpower lineup.

A month later, in June 1944, it had looked as though the longplanned institute might be getting underway. A senior trustee of the Wellcome Trust had indicated that a proposal for a medical research station in Egypt would receive favorable consideration.[8] Killearn thought that a representative from the Wellcome Trust should travel to Cairo to survey the situation and to formulate the conditions under which it could function in Egypt. He again warned Eden that there was no time to waste. If the Americans succeeded in defeating malaria, American prestige in Egypt would rise.[9] Despite Killearn's plea, however, neither the foreign office nor the Wellcome Trust took steps to establish the medical research institute in Cairo.

A year later, in the spring of 1945, Killearn learned that the Rockefeller campaign was indeed to be a success and that "every type of malaria" was being extinguished in Upper Egypt. He recalled that the "reputedly rather ferocious Dr. Soper" had personally told him that the Rockefeller Foundation "had no intention of tackling the normal malaria but only the pernicious breed."[10] Were the Americans stepping out of bounds? In July 1945 Eric Denholm Pridie, a British medical officer in the Sudan service who was visiting Egypt, assured Killearn that the malaria campaign had in fact been remarkably successful and that, without doubt, Egypt would soon owe the Rockefeller Foundation a debt of gratitude.[11]

Meanwhile, the rules of the game were changing. In 1945 Winston Churchill was voted out of office and a Labour government came to power. The Labour government believed its mission was to dismantle the empire and to redesign its postwar role in world affairs. The British people had suffered economic hardship in the postwar years and had been compelled to borrow $3.5 billion from the United States. Ernest Bevin, a former trade union leader and minister of labor from 1939 to 1945, who became foreign secretary, believed that his government should back moderate nationalist leaders in its imperial territories and give technical assistance in areas of social and economic reform. This form of involvement would maintain British influence through nonintervention; partnership would replace domination and prove an alternative means of preserving British power.[12]

Killearn was an imperialist at heart, but he agreed with Bevin on the importance of social and economic assistance as a means of retaining British influence. His belief in the importance of increasing British medical assistance was strengthened because the last British official in the Egyptian quarantine service had just lost his post.

Quarantines are of great political, commercial, and military significance because the quarantine administrators are able to survey and control entries and departures across international borders. Quarantines enable governments to survey and regulate civilian and military communications, commerce, and travel.[13] Few governments willingly cede their quarantine services to others. Under the terms of the 1936 Treaty between Egypt and Britain, British military forces had been exempted from Egyptian quarantine regulations in time of war. In World War II the agreement was extended to all Allied forces, including the French military after Vichy fell. The 1936 Treaty led to numerous violations of quarantine, which the Egyptians were powerless to stop. In December 1944, for example, pilgrims from Tunis to Mecca were being transported commercially via Cairo on a French military plane. The plane had made a stopover in Cairo, but because it was military it did not observe the quarantine regulations. Cholera had been transmitted to Egypt from outside more than once, and the Egyptian government was furious. The Egyptian Quarantine Administration protested to the French legation to no avail.[14]

British medical experts had long been stationed within the Egyptian quarantine service. In 1938 Britain and Egypt had agreed that a British official would serve in the Quarantine Administration as liaison between the Ministry of Health and British military authorities. The agreement was to expire on 31 October 1944.[15]

Khalil Abd al-Khaliq had decided not to renew the contract of the British official when the agreement expired. The British embassy requested that the decision be reconsidered because of the importance of unhindered Allied shipping through the Suez Canal and to and from Egyptian ports while the war was still on.[16] The Egyptian government nevertheless stuck to its decision and did not renew the contract.[17]

Killearn had hoped his British medical research institute could keep a "useful watch on quarantine developments" if there was no British doctor in the Egyptian quarantine service, but the plan had fallen through.[18] Now Killearn had decided that the appointment of a British medical expert to the British embassy was the best that could be done under the circumstances. That posting was one Killearn could manage since he had one such expert at hand: Dr. Pridie, the medical officer in Sudan.

In July 1945 Pridie was appointed health counselor to the British embassy in Cairo. He had worked in Sudan for many years and spoke Arabic fluently. His assignment was to strengthen the British medical connection in Egypt, to inspect and report on all health and medical activities, and to help Egypt with public health problems. At the time there was not a single British doctor in a responsible post in an Egyptian hospital or in the Ministry of Health's Quarantine Administration.[19]

Pridie began his new job in Egypt by preparing a memorandum outlining ways in which British medical research could compete with the Rockefeller Foundation. He thought steps had to be taken at once to establish a British medical research institute in Egypt. In general, he had found that medical research institutes had not been a success in the tropics because sooner or later they came into conflict with local authorities: in Egypt, he thought, it would be sooner rather than later. The Rockefeller Foundation had succeeded because it worked within the Ministry of Health. The British should follow suit and place British researchers in Egyptian research laboratories to "strengthen the British medical connection and forge a link unlikely to be affected by political intrigue or national prejudice."[20] He doubted if the Wellcome Trust would fund British researchers to work in Egyptian research facilities because it preferred to endow buildings that would carry its name. Nevertheless, something had to be done: every day of delay was a day lost to the British.[21]

Pridie then made a preliminary survey of the medical services of Egypt to see where British assistance might be needed. His survey reveals attitudes that were typical of British officials in Egypt in its patronizing tone and its lack of appreciation for the acute shortage of facilities, training programs, and funds for adequate salaries. In the survey, he stated that medical personnel failed in interpersonal relationships. Those in positions of authority lacked concern for their subordinates, while those suffering an injustice had no channels for appeal. The patient seldom complained if he were treated poorly by the orderly, and the orderly seldom complained if mistreated by the doctor, resulting in much abuse of authority. The low standard of honesty was a handicap for the scientist.[22] The quarantine service was, he decided, fairly efficient but suffered "from the subconscious tendency of the Egyptians to put foreigners to inconvenience" and to use the quarantine for political ends.[23] The Egyptian quarantine service officials often imposed excessive quarantine measures because, he said with some justification, they would be blamed if any disease broke out. He recommended that a small number of British doctors, nursing sisters, and medical researchers be recruited to reform the Egyptian medical services. He also thought the Egyptian government should hire a British professor of public health, and he concluded that the British must take steps to upgrade Egyptian medical services both to maintain the reputation of British medicine and to forestall the deterioration of public-health conditions. Otherwise, he predicted, the Egyptians would be forced to call in foreign experts to do what the British should have done.[24] He did not consider the years of British rule or the heritage of foreign political domination. He noted neither that Egyptian medical schools had long employed British professors of medicine nor that British nurses and medical researchers had worked in Egypt.

Meanwhile, foreign office officials in London were trying to find a means of accommodating expanding American interests. Ronald Campbell, who in 1945 was with the eastern department of the foreign office, prepared a memorandum on the deteriorating state of British-American relations in the Middle East. He thought that the British government intended to maintain its responsibility for defense of the Middle East and should welcome American assistance toward this end. He complained that the Americans had no regard for established interests and accused the British of wanting to exclude them. In truth, he asserted, the British welcomed cooperation in such projects as revising treaty arrangements with Egypt and defending the Suez Canal.[25]

The Americans, however, were less interested in giving assistance and cooperation than in establishing their own presence in Egypt. In the area of public health and medicine, the Rockefeller Foundation was especially active in trying to gain a permanent place in Egypt. Such men as Soper and Kerr assumed that the United States was destined to expand its role in the Middle East and that the British era was over. They believed that American scientific methods would improve the lot of poverty-stricken peoples and would thereby promote political stability. Just as Killearn suspected, Soper and Kerr had in early 1945 begun to try to convert their success in combating malaria into a more permanent establishment. First, Soper and Kerr had hoped to secure an invitation for the Rockefeller staff to reorganize the Epidemic Section of the Ministry of Health. Second, they had hoped to make Cairo the headquarters of the Rockefeller Foundation's Middle East division.

Egyptian ministry representatives had been unresponsive to initial inquiries, so Kerr again looked to the women from the Mabarra Muhammad Ali and Red Crescent for support. On 19 January 1945 the Mabarra women had invited the Rockefeller staff to a luncheon celebrating the Mabarra's first year of work in the field. They told the staff that they would continue their strong support of the Rockefeller work but would fight them if they did not approve of what they were doing.[26] The women had for some time been pressuring the ministry to invite them to stay on.[27] Kerr was pleased when some of the women from the Mabarra Muhammad Ali and the Red Crescent had asked him to demonstrate delousing procedures at the Huda Sha'rawi *izba* (estate), about ten miles from Cairo. He went with them to the *izba* and demonstrated how to use DDT louse powder against the body lice that carried both typhus and relapsing fever. On the way back to Cairo, the women told him that they would look to him for more help in the future. Kerr hoped they would use their influence with the Ministry of Health and would encourage it to develop an American-style delousing program to forestall future louse-borne epidemics.[28]

Kerr was well aware of British resentment of American activities in Egypt. When he learned of Pridie's appointment, he wondered if this was an attempt by the British to counteract American activities in public health. A colonel in the Royal Army Medical Corps had once told him that the Americans "had come into Egypt during the war and upset things a bit by the active work they had done."[29] Kerr concluded that Pridie was indeed a rival. His solution was to redouble his efforts to secure a greater role in the Egyptian public health service.

The British were soon to find competition from yet another American agency. When the war ended, the U.S.A. Typhus Commission had been disbanded, and the U.S. Navy's Bureau of Medicine and Surgery then offered to take over its facilities. In August 1945 Ali Tawfiq Shusha, the permanent secretary for health, agreed to the transfer of the U.S.A. Typhus Commission's facilities to U.S. Naval Epidemiological Unit 50. Nineteen its twenty-six Egyptian staff members were discharged from the U.S.A. Typhus Commission and were rehired by the U.S. Navy the following day. The remaining seven returned to the Giza Health Department. In October 1945 the epidemiological unit became the U.S. Naval Medical Research Unit 3 (NAMRU-3).[30]

Researchers at NAMRU-3 were to study epidemic diseases that could infect U.S. troops stationed in the Near East, Africa, and India. The unit would maintain small mobile teams that could immediately travel to the site of any outbreak of an epidemic disease. The navy stated that the laboratory would have only scientific (no political) objectives, but it was clearly a part of postwar American military expansion.

Faruq and the palace government, meanwhile, continued to emphasize the importance of public health. NAMRU-3 was to profit from this emphasis. In November 1945 Faruq had outlined a plan for public health reform "now that the war was over."[31] The government, he had announced, was allocating £E 25 million for potable water and improved sanitation in villages. Additional funds for new urban sanitation projects would be provided, and laws were being studied to limit land acquisition, to increase the number of small landowners, and to protect the tenants from the landlords.[32] In December 1945 Prime Minister Mahmud Fahmi al-Nuqrashi reiterated Faruq's promise that the government would allocate £E 25 million for the projects and £E 2 million for *birka* filling.[33] He then detailed the plans to upgrade water supplies, village sanitation, small village hospitals, and tuberculosis hospitals.[34]

Meanwhile, G. B. Dowling, the navy medical corp's representative, had arrived in Cairo to work out final arrangements. He learned that the minister of health, Ibrahim Abd al-Hadi, was away accompanying the *kiswa* (a black, embroidered tapestry made annually in Egypt and ceremonially transported to Mecca, where it was used to cover the *Kaʻba,* the focal point of the pilgrimage). Faruq, in announcing the selection of the minister of health to accompany the *kiswa,* said that this indicated that the health of his subjects was his greatest concern and that the budget of the Ministry of Health was being greatly increased. Dowling was encouraged to learn that public health had assumed a new political importance in Egypt. He thought that the government's having just granted Abd al-Rahim al-Dimirdash, director of the Fever Hospital at Abbasiyya adjacent to the NAMRU-3 compound, £E 65,000 for new hospital buildings boded well for the future of NAMRU-3.

Dowling's delegation received a warm reception from ministry officials, who insisted only that Egyptian researchers be attached to the unit. The Egyptians tried to play the Americans off against the British by authorizing a building site to which the British had rights, "but nothing came of it."[35] Shusha gave NAMRU-3 temporary permission to begin working, pending final negotiations. The secretary of the U.S. Navy officially recognized NAMRU-3 the following month, but political tensions prevented completion of the negotiations. A final agreement was delayed because Egyptian anti-British sentiment had suddenly been extended to Americans after Truman made a public statement in support of the Zionist claim to Palestine. When the American government supported the British position on Sudan, Egyptians were enraged. Suddenly Americans, too, found their cars stoned as they drove through town. In February 1946 during demonstrations called by the National Committee of Students and Workers, crowds attacked an American naval doctor walking in uniform.[36] NAMRU-3 officials realized that hostility toward the United States had increased and resolved to wait until conditions stabilized before working out the final agreement. In the meantime they were able to work with no obstacles.

From the first news of the project, British authorities were in a quandary. The United States had, of course, fought with Britain in the world war that had just ended. Immediately after having made the agreement with the U.S.A. Typhus Commission, Dowling had contacted the British naval medical liaison officer in Washington, D.C., to inform him of the plan. Dowling said he hoped for close cooperation with the British navy and other interested British organizations. The officer reminded his headquarters in London that in the invasion of Normandy Dowling had organized the U.S. Army's medical facilities. Dowling had insisted that he wanted "to avoid the slightest suggestion of an arbitrary American military incursion into a field which normally would be regarded as a British sphere of influence."[37] Yet this conclusion was inescapable.

Pridie was already wary of the American presence at the Abbasiyya Fever Hospital. In October 1945 while on a routine visit to the hospital, he had learned that researchers from the U.S.A. Typhus Commission were still there.[38] He did not yet know that the commission had just been taken over by the U.S. Navy. A month later when Dowling visited Egypt, he had immediately contacted Pridie to assure him that he was anxious to obtain full British cooperation. Pridie suspected that Dowling thought that the politically minded Egyptians might use the scheme to make trouble between the British and the Americans. Presumably with a straight face, he told Dowling that "medical research and politics had nothing to do with one another."[39]

Pridie then suggested that British and Egyptian researchers could work together with the Americans at NAMRU-3, and Dowling agreed. He reflected that this cooperation would make the research unit British, American, and Egyptian: a happy resolution.[40] The existence of NAMRU-3 would make it more difficult for the proposed British medical research institute, but, he rationalized, the Wellcome Institute had delayed making a decision for eighteen months. Even if the Wellcome Institute did come up with a plan to endow a medical research facility, it would be "considered as a counter-blast to the American proposal, which would be unfortunate."[41] Yet he was appalled at the thought of a complete American naval unit, with a minimum of sixteen officers and forty other ranks, stationed permanently in Cairo. He did not understand why it had to be military and not civilian, nor did he understand why the Americans could not carry out their research closer to home. He hoped the Egyptian government would drag its feet in coming to a decision on the proposal.[42]

Pridie was encouraged by an intimation from Shusha that American medical workers were not popular with Egyptian authorities and that Egypt was encouraging the project simply to be able to take over its equipment and facilities themselves. Pridie thought it best for the British to settle for the assignment of the British naval medical researchers to NAMRU-3 and then to concentrate on sending Egyptian researchers to British universities.[43] He was nevertheless dismayed when he learned that NAMRU-3 research workers intended to include India, which was still under British rule, in their terms of reference. He suspected that the Indian Medical Research Council would have views on that.[44]

Killearn, for his part, found his earlier predictions confirmed. He wrote Bevin that the Americans had beaten the British in the establishment of a medical research institute. He reminded Bevin that he had on more than one occasion urged an early British initiative in the field of medical research in Egypt. The British could not oppose the plan now that the Americans had gotten in first.[45] He thought that in view of Egypt's need for such an institute the British should not hamper the plan for political reasons but should rather make it the tripartite British-American-Egyptian concern Pridie had suggested. If the British held aloof, he suspected political reaction might go against them.[46]

The British Ministry of Health studied the matter and concluded that the proper British response to NAMRU-3 turned on the importance to the foreign office of maintaining British personnel in Egypt as a means of reinforcing British influence. The ministry felt it would be difficult to recruit British civilian personnel of the same caliber as the Americans, so the better course was probably the British-American-Egyptian approach. An unknown reader wrote, "no good, U.S. won't play" in the margin of the note.[47] But the United States did play. British research workers were eventually assigned to work at the research laboratory alongside the American and Egyptian personnel.[48]

In early 1946 Pridie reported that his mission was a success: on their own initiative Egyptian medical authorities in rural districts were beginning to consult him about health matters. He thought the success was attributable to the prestige of the British embassy there. Later he reported that he was being increasingly consulted about epidemics through unofficial, personal contacts.[49]

Pridie's mission fit in with the new postwar British foreign policy. Bevin thought that the British government should work to improve health standards in Egypt by eradicating the diseases transmitted by the Nile. The fellahin would be grateful for their improved well-being and would stop listening to the pashas, who continually blamed the British rather than themselves for Egypt's social ills. British-sponsored social and economic development would transform Egypt from an imperial dependency to an independent nation that would remain a partner in the British zone of influence.[50] Bevin may have been unwittingly replaying the conceits of Cromer, Gorst, and Kitchener, who had ruled Egypt before World War I. All three had believed that they were helping the downtrodden peasants against the undeserving and exploitative pashas and landowners. Egyptians of all classes, however, were demonstrating that they wanted not only national but also social and economic reform outside of any foreign zone of influence.

On 17 February 1946 in the wake of increasingly violent anti-British demonstrations and riots, Faruq appointed Ismail Sidqi prime minister. Sidqi came to power vowing to renegotiate the 1936 Treaty so that Egypt might win full independence from Britain and retain sovereignty over Sudan. Although he was unaffiliated with any political party, he was closely associated with the palace and with business and industrial interests and was considered a "strong man" who could restore order. He attempted with little success to quell the nationalistic demonstrations and riots and to suppress the active labor movement, which in a series of increasingly militant strikes, was calling for better working conditions and increased pay rates. He arrested and interned thousands of radical political activists and made their periodicals and other political materials illegal.

Perhaps in an effort to direct national attention to a less politically sensitive arena, he immediately announced a "War on Poverty, Disease, and Ignorance."[51] The government vowed to expand existing rural health centers, to undertake new potable water projects and nutrition and hygiene programs, to improve health propaganda, and to combat endemic diseases. In March the government established a committee to plan the projects.[52] In July 1946 Sidqi's Ministry of Agriculture announced that it would begin to study means of increasing the rural population's standard of living. The solution was to build rural social centers that would provide agricultural, social, and medical services. The rural social center project had originally been designed in 1939 by the Ministry of Social Affairs, which in 1941 had established eleven experimental centers for rural development. Now the government decided to expand the social centers, each of which was to serve ten thousand inhabitants.[53] At the end of the year in his annual speech from the throne, the king announced that the government would take all measures to curb disease and would establish new clinics, hospitals, and quarantine facilities in the southern and eastern areas of the country.[54]

Pridie observed that when Sidqi announced his war, he had made no mention of any sort of land reform, income distribution, or wage increases, nor had he mentioned that the population was rapidly increasing by a quarter million per year despite the high infant mortality rate of two hundred per thousand.[55] He thought that the increase in rural health centers proposed by Sidqi would at most be palliative and would not address the fundamental causes of poverty. Nevertheless, Pridie thought British medical personnel should be recruited to participate in the new programs. To that end he arranged an interview with Sulayman Azmi, a former dean of the Qasr al-Ayni Medical School who had been made the new minister of health. The meeting went well: Azmi said he was interested in utilizing British nursing sisters.[56] Sidqi then granted Pridie an interview. When Pridie asked him to allocate the money for British medical personnel, Sidqi laughed and said that "medicine was a question of humanity, not politics."[57] Pridie replied that there had been too much politics in the past. Later he reported that Sidqi's mind had not been on the meeting and that the purpose of the interview had been to "create an impression rather than to quench a sudden thirst for knowledge on public health and social conditions in Egypt."[58] Sidqi was presumably not relying on Pridie for information about public health and social conditions, rather he was seeking to further good relations with the British embassy. Despite Pridie's efforts, the British medical personnel were not hired.

Kerr also continued to hope for an increased role for the Rockefeller Foundation. He was impressed when Faruq announced the new allocation of funds because £E 25 million was many times its annual Ministry of Health budget and because the projects were the sort with which the Rockefeller Foundation could help.[59] Yet no invitation came. The change of government from Nuqrashi to Sidqi and the announcement of Sidqi's war on poverty, disease, and ignorance seemed auspicious for the Rockefeller Foundation's chances in Egypt because Amina Sidqi, one of its staunchest supporters, was the the new prime minister's daughter. She was the central figure in the Mabarra Muhammad Ali branch in Asiut, where she had been in close contact with the field headquarters of the Gambiae Eradication Service. When the Rockefeller Foundation had terminated its field office in Asiut, she had established a clinic in the vacated building.[60] She had earlier told Bruce Wilson, the Rockefeller Foundation's field director in Asiut, that the foundation should take charge of the Epidemic Section of the Ministry of Health and direct all control efforts in future epidemics.[61] Now Kerr hoped the Rockefeller Foundation would be invited to assist in Sidqi's war on poverty, disease, and ignorance. He jotted down five areas in which the Rockefeller Foundation might assist if asked.

1. Bilharzia. He would suggest implementing the program of snail destruction recommended by Rockefeller Foundation advisors in the Bilharzia Section of the Ministry of Health.

2. Nursing. He would recommend hiring an adequate staff of English-speaking nurses to teach in the school of nursing and hiring supervisors for the wards of Qasr al-Ayni Hospital, the largest public hospital in Cairo.

3. Tuberculosis. He would recommend establishing a tuberculosis hospital in Cairo where patients would be well cared for.

4. Medical Entomology Section. The Rockefeller Foundation could supply advisers for a new Medical Entomology Section.

5. Epidemic Section. The Rockefeller Foundation could assist in modernizing the methods of the Epidemic Section.[62]

Kerr proposed that his staff carry out a two-week survey and then submit formal recommendations to the ministry. He thought that even without the survey it was clear that ministry personnel should be better paid and that procurement procedures for supplies and equipment should be expedited. The new Epidemics Section should have the means to allow competent officials to handle serious emergencies so that extraordinary procedures would not be necessary in the future. He thought the best procedure would be to have a Rockefeller representative appointed special adviser to the undersecretary of the Ministry of Health.[63]

The competitors suddenly had a chance to prove themselves when an outbreak of relapsing fever reached crisis proportions in February and March 1946.[64] Relapsing fever, which was uncommon in Egypt and had not been seen for many years, had occasionally been diagnosed by malaria-control workers in 1944 and 1945, but now the disease was spreading quickly through Middle and Upper Egypt.[65]

Kerr and Pridie both hoped to give assistance during the relapsing fever campaign. For Kerr, the emergency seemed to present an ideal opportunity to test the ministry's training in the Rockefeller Foundation's methods of vector control. Louse control could be accomplished with a carefully planned and systematic delousing campaign, and DDT was available in large quantities. It was just the sort of campaign in which the Rockefeller Foundation specialized. Earlier, Soper in a speech on control methods to the Egyptian Medical Society, had outlined his procedures for delousing a large population, but they were not being used in early February 1946 when relapsing fever increased dramatically. Kerr had come to believe that bad public health administration alone prevented the ministry from utilizing modern methods in controlling the disease.[66] In touring stricken regions, he found that many people, including most women, refused to go to the DDT dusting stations to be deloused, so Kerr suggested that the Mabarra Muhammad Ali take over and dust families in their homes.[67]

King Faruq agreed. Remembering his role in the malaria epidemic and his association with the Mabarra Muhammad Ali and the Rockefeller Foundation, he took a personal interest in the relapsing fever epidemic. He had good reason for this interest. His popularity had slipped since 1944. News of his personal indiscretions percolated through the country, and the public was growing increasingly disgusted. While Sidqi's council of ministers was meeting to plan for the war against poverty, Faruq suddenly strode into the room and announced that he had come to claim the right of the poor to protection against disease and hunger. He urged the council to pass a law forcing landowners to improve the social conditions of their workers.[68] He then told the assembled ministers that the public health projects were urgently needed but that combating relapsing fever was even more urgent. Mobilization of all doctors and philanthropic organizations was needed. He informed the ministers that the Mabarra Muhammad Ali had already begun to organize relief.[69] The ministers replied that they would redouble their efforts to deal with Egypt's public-health problems.

The Muslim Brotherhood, a political organization that called for remaking Egyptian society according to Islamic law, also took a special interest in public health.[70] In 1943 Hasan al-Banna, who believed that public health was an essential component of Islamic social reform, had organized mobile units to help improve public health in villages and towns. The units cleaned streets and alleys, instructed people in the importance of cleanliness, performed minor first aid, and educated and encouraged people to use hospitals and to follow modern scientific medical procedures. The brotherhood also ran welfare and social services and called for reconstructing Egyptian villages and for training *umda*s to be civil servants who would preside over elected village councils.[71] In 1944 doctors belonging to the brotherhood began organizing free clinics and outpatient services. Members of the brotherhood, like other Islamic reformers, were consistent in their support for modern science and medicine and advocated the establishment of modern medical and public health facilities run according to Islamic laws.[72]

The organization was harshly critical of governmental promises of reform. When Sidqi made his announcement of his war on poverty, disease, and ignorance, *al-Nadhir,* a monthly magazine published by the Muslim Brotherhood, cynically predicted that the war would soon be forgotten. Disease, the journal said, was too important to too many people because it was a source of income for doctors, schools of medicine, pharmacists, health barbers, and orderlies. The epidemics gave the elite women of the Red Crescent, who dressed in the most fashionable uniforms and masqueraded as recruits in the war against poverty, the opportunity to get their pictures in the newspapers. *Al-Nadhir* categorically stated that poverty, disease, and ignorance were a result of hypocrisy. The reforms, according to the magazine, would be unnecessary if people would only practice their religious beliefs. If they eschewed greed and hypocrisy and gave the *zakat* (alms tax required by Islamic law) for social programs, the epidemics would not have occurred, and the war on poverty would not have been needed. Poverty, disease, and ignorance were challenges intended by God to provide an opportunity for Islamic reform.[73] Despite their critical attitude, members of the Muslim Brotherhood during the relapsing fever epidemic volunteered to assist the Ministry of Health in giving medical instruction and in organizing relief through their network of small clinics and dispensaries established throughout Egypt.[74]

Sulayman Azmi insisted that the ministry's control work was impeded by the popular belief that DDT was *haram* (forbidden). The volunteer women had, however, met with success in carrying out their delousing programs. When opposition senators attacked the government in Parliament for inattention to the epidemic, he said he would ask the women of the Mabarra Muhammad Ali and Red Crescent to expand their activities throughout Egypt.[75] The Red Crescent was assigned to Qina, Suhag, Fayum, Buhayra, Minufiyya, and Daqahliyya. The Mabarra was assigned to Asiut, Minya, Beni Suef, Giza, Qalyubiyya, Gharbiyya, and Sharqiyya. In each province the women organized a campaign against relapsing fever. The Egyptian army gave them transportation equipment.[76] While on tour in Upper Egypt, Azmi visited the women. In Minya he praised the women who had left their palaces to make life more tolerable for the needy by providing them with medicine and food. He praised the solidarity of men and women who worked together against the epidemic.[77]

Meanwhile, the ministry had exhausted its supply of DDT without

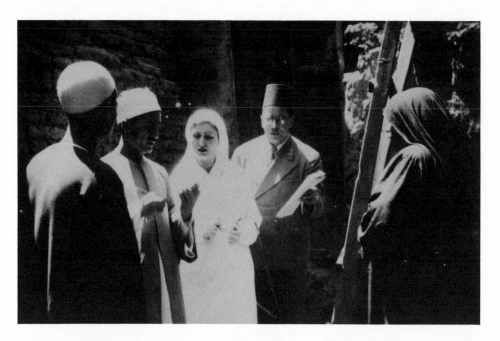

Fig. 12. Wadud Fayzi Musa, member of the Mabarra Muhammad Ali, making rounds during relapsing fever epidemic in Shabin al-Kum, March 1946. Courtesy of Wadud Fayzi Musa.

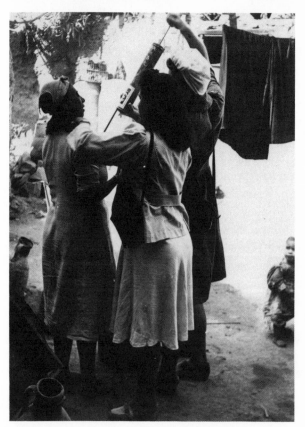

Fig. 13. Volunteer women disinfecting a fellahin woman with DDT. Source: USATC, RG 112, Box 67T, File 710, NA.

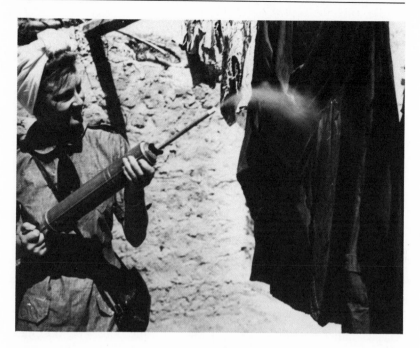

Fig. 14. Volunteer woman disinfecting clothing with DDT. Source: USATC, RG 112, Box 65T, File 710, NA.

affecting the spread of relapsing fever.[78] Sidqi then asked S. Pinckney Tuck, U.S. minister in Cairo, to assist in procuring some. Tuck agreed to release ten tons of DDT that the United States had stored in Egypt and to send another ten tons. Kerr arranged to send the insecticide by air because he thought support for Sidqi might be worth the high cost of airfreight.[79]

Less than a week after the American legation announced that it would supply the twenty tons of DDT, Pridie arranged for the British army to supply the Egyptian Ministry of Health with one hundred tons. A. M. Kamal, undersecretary for preventive medicine in the Ministry of Health and Egypt's foremost epidemiologist, said that he had known for some time that the British had large stores of DDT in Egypt. He had made repeated requests to Pridie and to British military authorities, but the British army would only release four tons, one ton at a time. Then, when the Americans made their offer and publicized it widely, the British army came through with five times the amount the Americans had offered.[80]

Armed with ample supplies of DDT, teams from the Ministry of Health rapidly expanded their delousing campaign. The Mabarra and Red Crescent women also disinfected persons in the stricken regions with DDT, injected acutely ill relapsing fever patients with Salvarsan to prevent death from myocarditis, and distributed relief supplies (figs. 12–14). The villages with rural social centers and health units proved to have very low infection rates because the medical personnel sprayed all homes and clothing without charge.[81] NAMRU-3 experts discovered that penicillin was effective in the treatment of the disease. Within a few weeks the disease was brought under control, and by mid-May 1946 relapsing fever had nearly disappeared.

In its report on the epidemic, the Ministry of Health stated that its system of control had been completely altered during the epidemic. It had substituted DDT for kerosene in its delousing procedures. It had treated the sick in their homes by using mobile units that toured the villages rather than by removing patients to infectious fever hospitals or to isolation camps. As a result, people hastened to report the disease, and "patients sought treatment having realised its value in effecting recovery."[82] The official number of cases from 1944 to 1946 was 128,541.[83] The official death toll from 1944 to 1946 was 3,295, but the actual figure was undoubtedly higher.[84]

Once again Khalil Abd al-Khaliq charged that the presence of British troops was responsible for the disease. He insisted that Egyptian workers with the Eighth Army had introduced the disease, which had broken out in North Africa in 1944.[85] A. M. Kamal disputed Abd al-Khaliq's thesis. He deduced from epidemiological analysis that the epidemic had been introduced through Suez, where men from Beni Suef worked. The workers had carried it home to Beni Suef, where it had first appeared, and it had spread throughout Middle and Upper Egypt.[86] Nevertheless, Abd al-Khaliq's charges further intensified the political nature of public health in the postwar era.

Killearn left Egypt in March 1946 for a post in Southeast Asia, feeling that he had been "kicked upstairs" in what he interpreted as a victory of the palace over the British embassy.[87] He was only partially correct, for his imperial style no longer represented British foreign policy. His successor, Ronald Campbell, tried to further Bevin's policy of retaining influence through partnership. Pridie continued to work on behalf of British medical interests in Egypt until 1949, when he retired to England. Kerr left Egypt in 1946, but Bruce Wilson and other Rockefeller Foundation experts and the NAMRU-3 researchers continued to work in Egypt.

In the postwar era bilateral technical assistance in public health and other fields had become an essential part of foreign policy. The American-British rivalry had further politicized public health in Egypt. Public health had become a complicated crusade in which the palace, the succession of governments, the radical opposition parties, and the big powers sought to prevail. The following year, the long-suffering nation was stricken by yet another epidemic. It was to have enormous and unprecedented political ramifications.

7

Cholera Goes out of Control

Al-Qurayn, a town in the date-producing district of Sharqiyya province, was located two miles from Tal al-Kabir, the largest British military base in Egypt, and five miles from Treaty Road (Tariq al-Mu'ahada), commemorating the 1936 Treaty with Britain (fig. 15). Twelve thousand people traveled each day from al-Qurayn to work at the base. Half of them had come from other regions of Egypt to find work. Since al-Qurayn's total population including the migrant workers was only twenty-one thousand, the importance of the military base in its economy was evident. Because of the relatively high salaries and the extensive smuggling from the base by Egyptian workers and their British accomplices, the town was enjoying a boom and was exceedingly, if temporarily, prosperous. In this respect it was different from any other town in Egypt.[1]

On 21 September 1947, an inhabitant of al-Qurayn had fallen ill with a mysterious disease and had died within hours. Dr. Sami Labib, director of al-Qurayn's hospital, was stumped. At first he suspected food poisoning because the man had severe vomiting and diarrhea. He sent samples from the man to Cairo for testing. The following day, ten more people fell ill with the mysterious disease. And in the evening, Dr. Labib had his answer: the disease was cholera.

Egyptian officials were entirely unprepared for an outbreak of cholera because Egypt's last epidemic of cholera had been in 1902. In 1947 it had become a distant memory associated with earlier days when

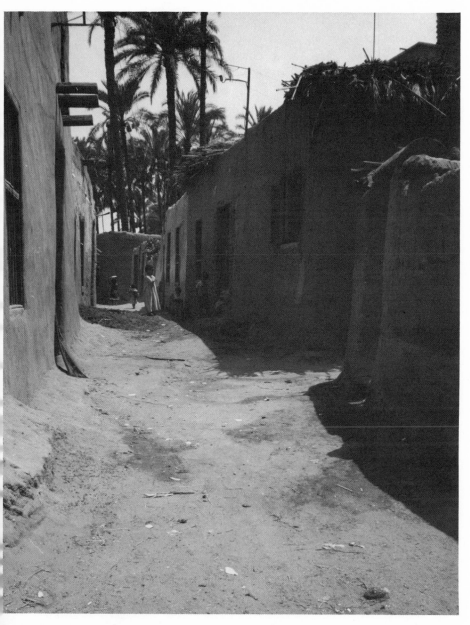

Fig. 15. A street in al-Qurayn, August 1983. Source: the author.

medicine and public health were far less advanced. The government, perhaps remembering the uproar caused by the Wafd government's hesitations and alleged concealment of the malaria epidemic only four years before, resolved with considerable fanfare to take all measures against the disease. In 1947 Egypt was once again ruled by Mahmud Fahmi al-Nuqrashi. Nuqrashi had returned to power in December 1946 following Sidqi's resignation over his failure to successfully renegotiate the 1936 Treaty and the total withdrawal of British troops. His was a minority government and knew it could not afford to fail against yet another natural disaster.

On 24 September Nagib Iskandar, the minister of health; Ali Tawfiq Shusha, permanent undersecretary of health; A. M. Kamal, director of preventive medicine; and Ismail Muhammad, director of immunology, departed for al-Qurayn. The minister of health, upon his return to Cairo, called a press conference. He announced that thirty-six new cases of cholera had appeared in al-Qurayn and the surrounding areas and urged the public to remain calm. Meanwhile, the army was ordered to surround al-Qurayn to prevent people from leaving, but the disease spread quickly.[2] A cartoon depicted the situation: the prime minister visits al-Qurayn and sees a sick man surrounded by soldiers. He asks their officer if the man is sick with cholera. No, the officer says, he is the only one who is not sick (fig. 16).

People in al-Qurayn soon felt like rats trapped in a cage. A new profession immediately developed: people smuggling. It cost twenty-five piasters to smuggle a person out of town. Smugglers helped people swim the canal, hid them in car trunks, or took them through the fields at night. Merchants in al-Qurayn to purchase dates also sneaked out of town carrying their wares with them. Of the twenty-two trucks that had been in the town before the epidemic, only four remained after the first week. The rest had gone through the cordon that according to one account leaked "like a sieve."[3] *Kashkul*, a propalace and anti-Wafd satirical journal, commented wryly that people fled following a *hadith* (Islamic saying or tradition): "flee the leper as you flee the lion."[4] Soon most of the towns on the Ismailia Canal, which was dug from the Nile to Suez to bring sweet water to canal workers, were infected.[5] British military authorities, citing the danger of cholera, promptly dismissed more than ten thousand Egyptian workers who were forced to leave

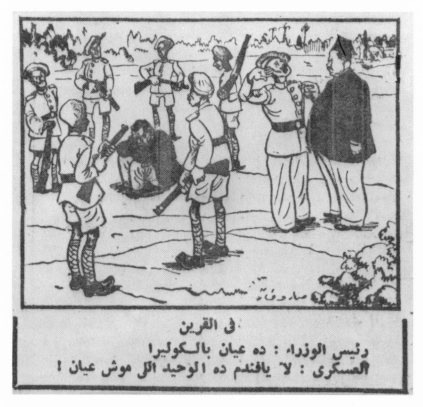

فى القرين :
رئيس الوزراء : ده عيان بالكوليرا
العسكرى : لأ يافندم ده الوحيد الّل موش عيان !

Fig. 16. In al-Qurayn, the prime minister says: "This must be a man sick with cholera." The soldier says: "No, *Effendi*, he is the only one who is not sick. Source: *Akhir Saʿa*, 29 October, 1947.

the bases and return to their homes.[6] Contacts between those leaving the infected region and the rest of Egypt were inevitable.

The Nuqrashi government now launched a war on cholera. Nagib Iskandar asked for a new account of £E 100,000 to combat the epidemic. Nuqrashi raised it to £E 500,000, the same amount ultimately allocated for malaria.[7]

A. M. Kamal set up a tent in Kafr Hamza, one of the worst hit areas, and stayed there throughout the epidemic to direct prevention and treatment procedures. A. M. Kamal, Muhammad al-Sayyid Umar, Anwar al-Mufti, and numerous other physicians and ministry officials worked with great dedication throughout the epidemic. They faced a daunting task. The lack of sanitation made transmission of the disease nearly unavoidable. In Habib Ayrout's words, if the fellahin do not have access to an artesian well or to the Nile itself, "they can only drink the brackish and stagnant water of the irrigation canals. Here men and animals cleanse and relieve themselves; vegetables, clothes and crockery are washed and carrion is thrown; and here the women come to get the 'drinking water.' Each fellaha (peasant woman) must bring back about six gallons for the next day's use. This water is added to what already remains in the *zir* (large clay pot) so that the bottom is never dry and never cleaned. The water stands all night, so that much of the dirt settles. It also cools, due to evaporation through the porous clay."[8] This was a system made for cholera transmission.

Akhir Sa'a, a weekly propalace magazine, published pictures of Evacuation Street (Shari'a Gala') in Cairo filled with garbage and scavengers.[9] *Akhbar al-Yawm* published a picture of fellahin filling their water cans with water from the Ismailia Canal despite ministry prohibitions.[10] Bruce Wilson received permission from the ministry to stay in the infected region where he could advise the ministry on control procedures.[11] Wilson was horrified at the lack of basic sanitation. In one section of the canal cordoned off by soldiers, he witnessed three men defecating in the canal, others bathing nearby, and still others washing cooking utensils.[12] When the Ministry of Health told the *umda*s to prevent people from drinking from the canals, the *umda*s replied that the people would then die of thirst. They had no other source of water.[13]

Local medical notions also contributed to the rapid spread of the disease. Rural people cut the air with wooden scissors to ward off the *jinn* (spirits) who, they believed, caused the disease (fig. 17). The *umda* of al-Qurayn told reporters that he predicted the disease would end because the birds of the town had returned, signaling the flight of the *jinn*.[14] Health barbers could only bleed their patients, cauterize them, or give them herbal remedies—all ineffective means of treating cholera.

Ministry officials, hoping to prevent transmission of the disease from person to person, ordered the isolation of all cases and contacts. The rural social centers formed committees that sprayed houses with DDT and cleared manure heaps. They placed barrels of disinfectant at the

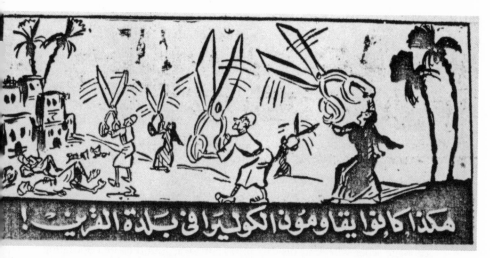

Fig. 17. "This is how they fight cholera in al-Qurayn." Source: *Ruz al-Yusuf,* 1 October 1947.

entrances to villages to disinfect vegetables and fruit. They installed 272 pumps for potable water at very short notice and vaccinated the inhabitants in their villages.[15] The Relief Section of the Ministry of Social Affairs set up a camp outside al-Qurayn where three thousand workers could be isolated under medical supervision until they could be returned to their homes.[16] In rural areas hospitals filled up, and patients were taken far from their families to be isolated in makeshift locations, which often lacked adequate sanitation. Fatality rates were over 50 percent. Wilson visited five isolation hospitals crowded with patients. The patients were covered with flies, but only one of the hospitals had been sprayed with DDT. Moribund cases were moved from their beds to the floor to make room for those who would live. He learned that the ministry was sending extra beds for those near death.[17]

The isolation of infected persons and their immediate families caused a violent reaction in many regions. The unfortunate victims were taken by the police to makeshift camps where they were interned in army tents. Escape attempts were frequent. Sa'id Abduh, a doctor who wrote articles about the epidemic, visited the isolation tents in al-Qurayn. He said well children were put in bed with their sick parents. People were terrorized by the appearance of the isolation teams. It was alarming, he said, for people to wake up in the morning and find their neighbor's house marked with a circle and a dot because it meant the isolation teams would come and take its inhabitants away.[18]

When panic reached dangerous levels, the ministry began to organize isolation camps in local school buildings nearer to people's homes. But people continued to conceal cases in fear of their being sent to the isolation camps. In Sharqiyya province the Ministry of Health heard a rumor that someone had died and that the family had tried to conceal it. Workers rushed to the village and found that the family had thrown the body down the well. It was too late; the disease had already spread.[19] In another village, police found a victim of cholera hidden in a canvas bag hung down a well, still alive.[20] In the most spectacular incident, which is still recalled today in conversations about the epidemic, a cabbage seller wheeling his cart into Cairo was found to be concealing under the cabbages the bodies of two men who had died of cholera. The man was arrested and his cargo impounded (fig. 18).[21]

A noted Egyptian novelist, Andree Chedid, in her novel about the 1947 cholera epidemic entitled *The Sixth Day,* captured the attitudes of many rural people to the isolation camps.[22] In it, an elderly woman named Um Hasan, upon learning that cholera had ravaged her village, felt compelled to leave Cairo where she had lived for many years to search for her relatives. When she arrived in the village, she found the houses empty and dark, crushed under piles of branches and straw. The interior had been burned by the medical police. Suddenly she encountered a nephew who told her of the epidemic's ravages.

"People in the towns don't get cholera," he said. "It's only for us. . . . We've had eleven deaths in our family. As for the village, I've lost count. But the hospital is the worst! The ambulance arrived, the nurses forced their way into the houses, burnt out belongings, carried off the sick."

"Where to?" the aunt asked her nephew.

"They never tell us. I found out in the end where they had taken my father and brother: under tents, right out in the desert. I've been there. At first they chased us away with sticks, my mother and me, but we returned shouting out the names of our people, so that they should know we hadn't deserted them, that we were there, near them. In the end I crept into one of the tents. It was horrible! The same face everywhere: blue, hollow, the tongue hanging out. The patients lie one

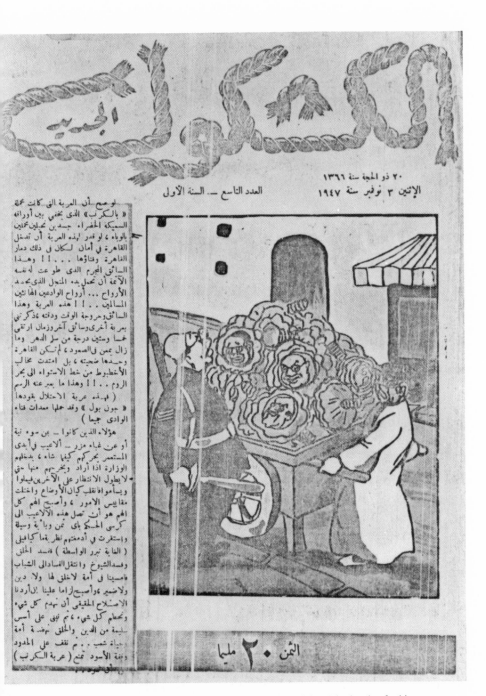

Fig. 18. A vendor is pushing his cart full of cabbages into Cairo. The heads of cabbages are party leaders. Source: *Kashkul,* 3 November 1947.

beside the other on the sand, vomiting; two of them were already dead and left lying there. I called again, they all looked at me in a dazed way. A nurse came in wearing boots and a mask, he pushed me outside—before I could find my people. No one who hasn't lived through all this knows anything about it. Never shall I forget—Since then we've hidden our sick and even our dead!"[23]

All over Lower Egypt people from the poorer classes were forced into isolation camps. Their anger and resentment increased until they began attacking their guards. In one instance, troops had fired on canal boatmen who were trying to evade a cordon near Alexandria.[24] The restrictions on travel and the marketing of produce had threatened the livelihood of persons in the infected region. The inhabitants of al-Rashid (Rosetta), a town on the Mediterranean, had stoned an ambulance carrying suspected cases of cholera to a government hospital.[25] The following day, near Alexandria, more than a thousand inmates trying to escape an isolation camp stoned police guards. The army was called in to restore order. In Buhayra inmates burned the tents of their isolation center. One reporter wrote that people cursed their relatives who caused them this trouble. Another said she was happy in the camp because she ate meat and vegetables rather than beans and radishes.[26] Hers was a minority opinion.

Indigenous political organizations also rushed to help. At the first news of the epidemic, the Muslim Brotherhood volunteered to help. One of its newspapers announced that forty thousand of its best youth from all over the Nile Valley had volunteered to assume their share of responsibility in curbing the epidemic. According to the newspaper, the volunteers were thoroughly committed, well disciplined, and well supervised in everything they did. They offered to distribute leaflets issued by the Ministry of Health, to help people understand them, to care for patients, and to help in cordoning the infected areas. Cholera was an enemy, the newspaper declared, and the Muslim Brotherhood was capable of fighting it. The Students' Section of the General Headquarters of the Muslim Brotherhood sent a letter to the Ministry of Health declaring the readiness of thousands of its members to curb cholera by whatever means it suggested.[27] The brotherhood formed a cholera control administration which claimed to have organized five hundred locals. Teams drove through the streets in a truck with a loudspeaker instructing people about health regulations. Its weekly journal asked its readers to follow the Ministry of Health's recommendations and carried articles reporting the latest cholera research by Leonard Rogers, a British cholera expert.[28]

Members of Young Egypt formed a committee to fight cholera in Sharqiyya province, where they placed themselves at the disposal of the Ministry of Health.[29] The committee organized teams to go the mosques to explain how to fight cholera and to discuss the role of the British in causing the epidemic.[30] Ahmad Husayn, president of Young Egypt, called on every member to make himself a soldier against cholera, to spread correct health principles among people, to teach methods of resistance, to organize assistance, and to lead the campaign through local committees on every street, village, *izba,* and town. In this way they would turn the disaster into an opportunity to organize and to develop social cohesion. Members of Young Egypt, he concluded, should encourage people to cooperate with the Ministry of Health.[31] In Damanhur, capital of Buhayra province, twenty-three volunteers from Young Egypt registered themselves with the Ministry of Health. Toward the end of October at its headquarters, the organization formed the General Committee to Fight Cholera. At the meeting, Abbas al-Aswani, a noted poet, spoke about the efforts of the government and the need for action. Fakhri Asad, a Coptic physician, was named head of the committee. He organized health propaganda against cholera.[32] Ibrahim Shukri, the vice president of Young Egypt, went to his village, Izba Mahmud Basha Shukri, in Daqahliyya province, to fight cholera. People there told him to go back, but he refused and proceeded to organize the campaign against cholera, which had been brought to the village by migrant (*tarahil*) workers. Ibrahim Shukri had the fellahin injected with anticholera vaccine and had the sick isolated. Six *tarahil* had died before he arrived, but there were no further deaths after his control effort began.[33]

Makram Ebeid, the leader of the opposition Kutla party, announced that the party's newspaper would participate in the epidemic by publishing any and all complaints against the Ministry of Health.[34] The Wafdist newspaper *al-Balagh* complained that the Nuqrashi government had refused to let its reporters into the stricken area, so they were unable to witness any deficiencies in procedure. In Cairo, however, workers were demonstrating against government negligence. According to the newspaper, a worker at the Sibahi factory near Shubra al-Khayma, an industrial suburb of Cairo, was stricken with cholera in the morning and waited in vain for an ambulance until his companions carried him away that evening themselves.[35]

The Wafd party formed a committee to study the cholera crisis and published a report on the government's shortcomings in dealing with the epidemic.[36] The report focused on weaknesses in containing the disease and claimed that the Wafd government had contained malaria in Aswan and Qina and had kept the death rate at 8 percent. The report recommended that the Wafdist youth organization should form teams under the supervision of Wafdist doctors. The teams would vaccinate people, visit hospitals and isolation camps, report on any problems, and collect statistics because the government statistics were not correct.[37] The last week of October, one thousand Wafd youths volunteered to help in al-Munira, a Wafdist stronghold that had been badly stricken with cholera.[38]

Haditu, the communist coalition, formed several Egyptian Students' Associations to Fight Cholera to assist people in the poorer quarters of Cairo.[39] The associations opened locals in Sayyida Zaynab, Bab al-Luq, Bulaq, Imam Shafi, Abbasiyya, Giza, Shubra, and Rod al-Farag— all quarters or suburbs of Cairo. They also operated in Alexandria and elsewhere. The Sudanese Committee for Cholera Control, composed of sixty Sudanese youths, worked with the Egyptians. The associations organized phenol units, which distributed soap, phenol, and lysol. They reported suspected cases, put voluntary quarantines around them, and waited with the sick until the doctor came. Haditu wrote that the masses must be organized into units headed by thousands of revolutionary leaders.[40] The Egyptian Students' Associations to Fight Cholera were to be prototypes for these organizations. Haditu then called on the government to take steps to make available purified water, phenol, soap, gasoline, and DDT to the poor who could not afford them. The government, Haditu suggested, should impose an "epidemic tax" to pay for the supplies.[41]

The Ministry of Health refused to work with the "political students," saying that the situation was under control.[42] After about two weeks of operations, police began breaking up Haditu's associations and arresting and jailing participants. The Muslim Brotherhood sent thugs armed with clubs to attack the communist locals. Haditu claimed that the secret police were acting as agents provocateurs, instigating violence to justify police repression. It further claimed that the police allowed the Muslim Brotherhood to circulate in a truck with a loudspeaker, while Haditu was allowed only a truck and a bullhorn to make its announcements. Finally, Haditu reported that the police had disbanded the locals and arrested many of the participants.[43] The current government did not want help from its opponents during the cholera epidemic any more than the Wafd government had wanted help from its opponents during the malaria epidemic.

Meanwhile, the Ministry of Health had decided to have the entire population of Egypt vaccinated with anitcholera vaccine to prevent it from spreading throughout Lower Egypt and into Upper Egypt. Since cholera was not a disease endemic in Egypt, nor was it anticipated by Egyptian medical officials, the supply of vaccine on hand had been very limited. At the first news of the outbreak, Nagib Iskandar had contacted the commander of NAMRU-3, Captain E. A. Phillips, for assistance in procuring the needed vaccine.

It was a golden opportunity for Phillips and for NAMRU-3, which was still operating without an official agreement. During the war, Phillips had worked with the U.S.A. Typhus Commission in Cairo. When the war ended and the U.S. Navy took over the commission's facilities, Phillips enlisted and in June 1947 had returned to Cairo to take command of the unit. Before the war he had participated in a project to determine the specific gravity of blood to facilitate blood transfusion for the war wounded. Knowledge gained in this project was to aid greatly in the treatment of cholera in Egypt.[44] NAMRU-3 had the means of procuring the anticholera vaccine.

Phillips wired naval officials in Washington, D.C., to rush the vaccine to Egypt. On 25 September the first U.S. Navy airplane left the United States with the ten thousand pounds of medical supplies requested by NAMRU-3. Four other planes flew additional supplies, stopping only to unload the shipment in Cairo. The crews had not had time to get visas and to clear quarantine controls, so they were not allowed to enter, pointedly demonstrating their adherence to Egyptian quarantine controls.[45] When the vaccine arrived, it was taken to NAMRU-3, where personnel from the adjacent Abbasiyya Fever Hospital began vaccinating all comers. Long lines formed outside the unit. The U.S. government eventually sent enough vaccine for six million people. The American consul general in Alexandria asked the embassy in Cairo to obtain and distribute anticholera vaccine, arguing that this action would render public service, relieve anxiety, and create goodwill all at the same time.[46] American officials hoped the vaccine airlift had helped in counteracting the anti-American feeling that arose following the U.S. government's support of Britain when the United Nations took up the Anglo-Egyptian dispute over the future of Sudan.[47]

During the first two weeks of the epidemic, the Egyptian press was full of news about American vaccine shipments being unloaded at Almaza Airport outside Cairo. The Arabic-, French-, and English-language presses in Egypt all wrote approvingly of the American response. One even called it "one of most spectacular examples of medical cooperation in history."[48] The gratitude expressed in the press was not entirely spontaneous. The American embassy's press attaché forwarded the clippings to the navy's public relations division, explaining that the "Thank You America" editorials were collected from a group of ten articles written by the U.S. Information Service editor at his office. Most of the photographs were also issued by the information service at the request of ten Egyptian newspapers.[49]

Such publicity was the order of the day. It was a time of international scientific cooperation and rapid medical advance. In the postwar years it was widely believed that medicine and science alone could unite the world. A friend of Bess Truman, wife of President Harry S. Truman, sent her a newspaper clipping, an editorial written by the editor of the *Journal d'Egypte*. She asked that Mrs. Truman place the editorial on the president's desk. It claimed that the "front" against the cholera bacillus had formed as rapidly as the bacillus had attacked. Nations around the world had mobilized their resources to send vaccine and sulfa drugs to Egypt. It asked whether it would not be possible to unite in a similar effort to destroy the atomic bomb.[50] The editorial expressed the pro-science spirit of the times and the hope that international humanitarian cooperation could break down political barriers.

British laboratories also rushed cholera vaccine to Egypt. The *Egyptian Mail*, a newspaper put out for British troops, wrote that despite current political differences there was underlying friendly feeling between Britain and Egypt and that the people of Britain were delighted to help a friend in need.[51] The British government donated 1.4 million doses of cholera vaccine, and British pharmaceutical companies sold 1.8 million doses to the Egyptian government.[52] Payment was deducted from funds the British government had owed the Egyptian government since the war. Meanwhile the British embassy informed the foreign office that it had a number of surplus ambulances in Egypt that were unsalable. A gift of the ambulances would "not be without further effect on British interests and our own future interests here."[53] The British government donated 12 ambulances, loaned 25, and sold 25 on terms favorable to the Egyptian government.[54]

Pridie was unable to participate in the first weeks of the cholera outbreak because he was vacationing in the United States. He was touring the Grand Canyon when he read about the cholera epidemic in a Sunday newspaper. He immediately returned by air to Cairo, where he found the Egyptian government had taken all measures possible against the spread of the "very unexpected and alarming outbreak."[55] Pridie then coordinated British relief efforts, inspected Egyptian control methods, and aided John Taylor and Bruce White, cholera experts sent by the National Institute for Medical Research.

The World Health Organization (see pp. 152–53) proved its merit during the cholera epidemic, which was its first major public-health crisis. In a massive undertaking, its officials combed pharmaceutical laboratories around the world for cholera vaccine, arranged for discounted prices to be paid by the Egyptian government, and coordinated production and shipment of thirty-two tons of vaccine to Egypt.[56] Under direction from the WHO, laboratories in Bombay worked overtime to prepare the vaccine for Egypt. India sent three million units of vaccine. The Soviet Union donated a million units.[57] Iraq, Syria, and Lebanon sent vaccine and medical missions. Italy, Switzerland, Holland, Sweden, France, and Denmark all sent needed supplies. The Turkish government sent five hundred thousand units of vaccine, and the Turkish Red Crescent sent a medical team assisted by Lutfiya Shawkat, daughter of former Khedive Abbas Hilmi (r. 1892–1914). She acted as nurse and interpreter for the Turkish medical team that assisted at the Abbasiyya Fever Hospital.[58] The Suez Canal Company attempted to vaccinate all persons in the Ismailia region.[59] The Mufti of Jerusalem Amin al-Hussayni, then in exile in Cairo, recruited a team of Palestinian doctors to help during the cholera epidemic.[60]

Judah Magnes, president of Hebrew University, Jerusalem, sent a letter to the Egyptian government, saying that Hadassah, the Women's Zionist Organization of America, had arranged with the university to send vaccines and Jewish doctors to Egypt. However, *al-Ahram* reported that Hebrew University wanted Egypt to send a plane with a sample of the microbe so that the university could prepare a vaccine.[61] Egyptians suspected that his offer was an indirect means of forcing them to recognize the Zionist presence in Palestine and therefore did not act on it. The *New York Times,* in an editorial entitled "Mercy and Fanaticism," wrote that it was "incredible that racial and political fanaticism could rise so high as to refuse medical aid even from an unwelcome quarter in the midst of a raging epidemic. . . . What a splendid victory for the Arab League!"[62] *Akhbar al-Yawm* bitterly attacked the *New York Times* coverage, claiming that the Zionist lobby was trying to defame Egypt. The Egyptian government, it pointed out, had accepted assistance from nations around the world. The newspaper angrily stated that it was not reasonable to demand that Egypt accept the entry of the Zionists who "threatened to destroy its cities under the guise of being messengers of humanitarianism."[63] This was the only offer that required an Egyptian plane to carry a sample of the vaccine to the donor and the only offer it did not accept.

The Republic of China sent a vaccine prepared in the Biological and Chemical Institute of the Ministry of Health in Shanghai. U.S. military aircraft then transported the Chinese vaccine. The American embassy arranged for a photograph of Iskander and Shusha, thanking both the Chinese legation and the American Air Force commander for the vaccine airlift. The American embassy's press attaché complained that the air force's publicity had played into the theme of "American imperialism" because it advertised the strong American military presence in China while the Republic of China's role had been underplayed.[64]

Amidst unprecedented publicity airplane after airplane landed in Cairo, where boxes of vaccine were unloaded and distributed to vaccination centers. Ministry officials then had to sort out the vaccines, which varied considerably in strength and quality. Ministry laboratories made a display of the vaccines, which ranged "from a slightly turbid suspension to a sort of *crème de vibrions*—of which the Soviets afforded the extreme example."[65] The ministry believed that the most reliable vaccines came from the United States, Britain, and India, so they were used in the cholera-stricken regions of Lower Egypt. Meanwhile Egyptian laboratories at Agouza were working around the clock making a vaccine, and by mid-October Egypt was nearly self-sufficient. The Ministry of Health organized teams to vaccinate the millions of people who lived near the infected regions and then the rest of the nearly twenty million Egyptians. *Al-Assas,* published by the ruling Sa'dist party, proudly announced that Egypt was the first nation to undertake a general vaccination of its entire population.[66]

The ministry's task was compounded by the popularity of vaccination. Bruce Wilson visited Faqus, one of the first towns where cholera had appeared, on a day when "16,000 of its 10,000 inhabitants" had showed up for vaccination![67] He learned that the extra six thousand were partly people who had already shown up for one shot and, just to be safe, had returned the same day for a second shot and partly people from the surrounding towns.[68] There was no sign of a fatalistic stance toward epidemic disease or of popular resistance to preventive vaccination and modern medicine during the 1947 cholera epidemic.

Wilson had immediately offered the Rockefeller Foundation's assistance in the cholera emergency. Ali Tawfiq Shusha, the permanent undersecretary of the Ministry of Health, welcomed the offer and asked Wilson and John Weir, a Rockefeller staff member who had taken Kerr's place in 1946, to act in an advisory capacity. Wilson organized an antifly campaign and moved to the infected zone for the duration of the epidemic. Weir stayed in Cairo, where he acted as advisor for the new fly-destruction program. The two organized a fleet of airplanes to spray Cairo and its suburbs with insecticide in hopes of reducing its fly population. Wilson wrote the head office in New York that the informal arrangement would not give the Rockefeller Foundation's International Health Division the official position it merited but hoped it was acceptable since it was temporary.[69]

Soon Royal Egyptian Air Force and U.S. Army pilots were spraying towns and cities from the air. The ten Egyptian pilots became known as the Faruq Health Squadron. Inhabitants of Cairo remember being instructed to stay indoors with their windows open while the planes flew overhead spraying what one recalls was "an intensive bombard-ment with DDT."[70] And within hours, the fly population decreased dramatically. A NAMRU-3 staff member designed a device for spraying DDT from a jeep, and soon a NAMRU-3 crew was going through towns and villages spraying streets and houses. After three days, how-ever, the fly population had returned to previous levels. Wilson was forced to conclude that the antifly campaign had been a failure. There were simply too many flies and the insecticide could not reach all of them.[71]

The Rockefeller staff followed a policy of avoiding publicity because of the sensitivities of the Ministry of Health, repeatedly turning down requests for interviews from the local and international media. Mean-while the American embassy was issuing daily press releases on the contribution of NAMRU-3's approach to public relations, but he felt that the Rockefeller policy of avoiding publicity would pay off in the long run.[72]

From the start Egypt's cholera epidemic was international news. Fear of the epidemic led many nations to cut trade and communication with Egypt. Iran, Italy, France, and Greece refused to admit all persons traveling from Egypt. Saudi Arabia placed travelers from Egypt in a five-day quarantine. France impounded all mail from Egypt for an in-definite period.[73] Shusha called such restrictive measures "cholera hys-teria" and complained that countries that stopped importing Egyptian cotton or that refused mail from Egypt were following a "quarantine of the jungle."[74] He asked the World Health Organization to monitor Egypt's control procedures. In October the World Health Organization held a special meeting to discuss conditions in Egypt and to coordinate international quarantine procedures. Muhammad Nazif, Egypt's new undersecretary of health for the Quarantine Administration, flew to Geneva and gave a summary of the measures the Egyptian Ministry of Health was taking to control the epidemic. The organization decided the measures were adequate and in accord with international health guidelines but recommended that Cairo and Alexandria be declared infected areas, which was promptly done.[75] It sent two experts, P. M. Kaul, director of the organization's Epidemiological Intelligence Sta-tion in Singapore, and W. W. Yung, director of the Department of

Epidemic Prevention, National Health Administration, Nanking, China, to advise the government on methods that had been used to control cholera in India and China. The organization then recommended that overzealous and unnecessary quarantine measures be dropped to prevent total disruption of Egyptian international relations, and the quarantines were gradually lifted.

On 10 October the ministry announced that there were still fewer than ten thousand cholera cases, but no one believed the daily reports. Even *al-Musawwar,* a propalace publication, thought the real figure was at least five times higher.[76] Indeed, government authorities admitted privately that the figure was much higher than ten thousand cases. That figure had been based on the number of cases taken to isolation, admittedly only a portion of the total. The ministry was growing desperate because despite its energetic measures the disease was still spreading. It now threatened to invade Upper Egypt, where a few isolated cases had already appeared. Because of the population's general failure to notify the ministry about cases, the government raised the penalty for nonnotificaion. Nagib Iskandar on 18 October announced that all travel from Lower to Upper Egypt, travel from one province to another in Lower Egypt, and navigation on the Nile and its branches were prohibited. The Egyptian air force was sent to clean the streets of Cairo. All leaves were canceled for the thirteen hundred Egyptian army troops working with the Ministry of Health.[77]

In response to the worsening crisis the Egyptian Ministry of Health stepped up its efforts to contain the disease. Trains on the Port Said–Cairo route were ordered not to stop at stations along the Ismailia canal. Boats were prevented from traveling on the canal. When the epidemic began, about seven thousand Egyptian pilgrims had left for Mecca, long a center of cholera transmission. The government prevented the rest from leaving and carefully monitored the returning pilgrims.[78]

The government also delayed the opening of parliament, schools, and universities.[79] It announced that the Egyptian army would not play a major role in the contemplated Arab invasion of Palestine because Egyptian troops were engaged in cordoning off the infected areas.[80] The opposition immediately jumped on such announcements. The Wafdist newspapers claimed that the government was afraid to face the country.[81] *Al-Kutla,* the newspaper of Makram Ebeid's party, said that cholera had come to Nuqrashi's rescue, just in time to keep him from resigning after his failure to win support for Egypt's case at the United Nations.[82] Regardless of such commentary the epidemic was a genuinely serious emergency. The intense governmental actions to combat it were not intended to cover up other failures but to avoid an even more serious emergency.

Despite the restrictions on travel, thousands of Cairo's inhabitants, living in the poorest neighborhoods, were soon infected with the disease. Cholera was the talk of the day. Journalists interviewed ordinary people, asking them their opinion about the disease. One old man said it was all a British plot to divert people from asking them to leave Egypt. Another, a peddler, said that the Ministry of Health urged people to keep flies away because they transmit cholera, but, he reasoned, if flies transmitted cholera they would have died since they are much weaker than human beings. Others thought it was a conspiracy so that Egyptians could not travel to attend sessions of the Security Council at the United Nations, where they were to be "sentenced in absentia."[83] Such conspiracy theories abounded.

Enterprising businesses eagerly commercialized the epidemic. Zama Company of Zamalek announced that its cognac drunk regularly would protect against cholera; because of the expected demand, customers were limited to two cases apiece. A restaurant on Elfi Street advertised that famous doctors patronized it during the epidemic because of its cleanliness. Cinema Metro announced a film about the beginning and end of the nuclear bomb; all proceedings of the first showing would go to help victims of cholera.[84] As cholera spread out of control the imam of al-Azhar mosque recited a *du'a* (supplication to Allah) for deliverance from the disease.[85]

Badrawi Ashur, a wealthy businessman and Fuad Sirag al-Din's father-in-law, visited the Egyptian government's Serum Institute. According to *Akhir Sa'a* and *Kashkul,* he had promised to donate £E 40,000 for a new wing for the institute but had later reneged on the promise. *Akhir Sa'a* calculated that Badrawi Ashur earned about £E 0.4 million in interest per year on his land and assets, so according to the *zakat* of 10 percent, he owed £E 40,000 for public welfare because he had given nothing.[86] *Kashkul* contrasted Badrawi Ashur with

Mr. Avierino, a Greek department store owner who had loaned one hundred trucks and five hundred tents to be used in the cholera-control effort, and with a Greek widow, who had donated a quarter of her inheritance to the campaign. The widow said that when her husband had immigrated to Egypt he had been penniless. In Egypt he had become wealthy, so she wanted to give part of it back to the people. Thus, while foreigners had been generous during the epidemic, wealthy native Egyptians like Badrawi Ashur, *Kashkul* argued, had not been generous and should be tried in court.[87] Many of Egypt's wealthy elite, however, did volunteer to assist during the epidemic.

Ahmad Lutfi al-Sayyid, the rector of Fuad I University, headed the General Committee to Aid Cholera Victims in Daqahliyya province. In a meeting in al-Mansura, he called on notables from Daqahliyya living in Cairo to return to their villages to help in the control effort. The committee collected donations for the Red Crescent and the Mabarra.[88] By the first week of November the wealthy had donated substantially to the benevolent societies and to the government programs for organized relief.[89]

In mid-October the Ministry of Health had asked the women of the Mabarra Muhammad Ali and the Red Crescent for assistance. The two benevolent societies had established vaccination centers in towns the ministry assigned to them throughout Lower and Upper Egypt. Princess Fawziyya, who had replaced Princess Chevikar as head of the Mabarra, announced that King Faruq had asked the organization to collect funds and supplies for distribution to the stricken people.[90] When the ministry burned the clothes of inmates in isolation camps, the Red Crescent and the Mabarra distributed new clothes. Relief workers in the infected provinces collected money and clothing, which they gave to the Red Crescent and the Mabarra Muhammad Ali for distribution to the cholera victims.[91] Hidiya Afifi Barakat, organizer of the Mabarra, was featured on the cover of *al-Musawwar,* distributing clothes to the needy.[92] Mary Kahil worked in the Abbasiyya Fever Hospital. The organization expanded during the epidemic and opened a new branch in Minya, which vaccinated eighty-five thousand persons and distributed food, clothing, and financial aid. Altogether the women established fourteen new vaccination centers where several hundred thousand people were vaccinated. The Women's Committee of the Red Crescent organized committees to visit houses in poor neighborhoods to give advice in curbing the epidemic. By early November the Red Crescent teams had vaccinated 51,393 persons.[93] The epidemic peaked on 31 October, when more than eight hundred new cases were reported by the isolation centers. In an effort to tighten procedures, the Ministry of Health announced that *umda*s of infected villages would be dismissed and prosecuted if three or more people died of cholera per week outside the isolation camp of their village. The government prosecuted 117 *umda*s, dismissed six of them, and fined the rest.[94]

In early November cholera finally began to abate. The remaining inmates in the camp at al-Qurayn were given small sums of money and sent home.[95] By the end of that month very few cases remained in the Delta. In early December a few cases broke out in Fayum, but by the middle of the month the Ministry of Health concluded that the epidemic was over. The last case was declared on 31 December 1947 in Cairo.[96] Egypt breathed a sigh of relief, and Nagib Iskandar posed for a triumphant photograph with the women volunteers (fig. 19). The disease had been contained before it had established itself in the major cities and before it had spread to the rest of the country.

The epidemic was officially and symbolically declared over on 11 February 1948, Faruq's birthday, exactly four years after his trip to Upper Egypt to visit the malaria victims. It had actually lasted about ten weeks, from the end of September to early December 1947.[97] At least 2,270 towns and villages had been stricken with the disease. Ministry of Health officials congratulated themselves: mortality had been one-seventh that of Egypt's 1902 epidemic. It was the first time in history that a cholera epidemic, spreading at the rate of a thousand new cases per day, had been controlled within six weeks. Not a single case had spread outside Egypt.[98]

A. M. Kamal, director of preventive medicine, went over the official records and adjusted the final statistics to 23,638 cases and 11,755 deaths. Ministry officials subsequently concluded that there were at least thirty-five thousand cases and about twenty thousand deaths.[99] Kamal later made an extensive study of the epidemic and became known as the "father of epidemiology" in modern Egypt. *Epidemiology of Communicable Diseases,* in which he wrote the chapter on cholera, was to become a standard reference for Egyptian students specializing in public health.[100]

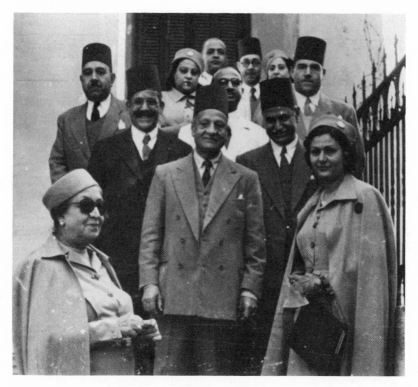

Fig. 19. Nagib Iskandar (center), the minister of health, and volunteers just after the cholera epidemic waned. Courtesy of Wadud Fayzi Musa.

Cholera experts sought to learn which aspects of the control process had been effective. Efforts at improving sanitation were judged to have been too limited to have been of use, and it was not clear if the mass vaccination had helped. A. M. Kamal thought that the vaccination program had not been effective because the disease had been transmitted too rapidly for vaccinated persons to have built up immunity after the vaccine. In his view, vaccination had done more harm than good because the ministry had not had the means of sterilizing the syringes. In consequence, many cases of hepatitis had followed the mass vaccination. He later concluded that the greatest achievement of the control effort had been in shielding Upper Egypt by stopping all traffic for ten days. The "escapees and stampeders" from the infected region, many of whom were carrying or incubating the disease, were prevented from spreading the disease any further than Lower Egypt.[101] In consequence, only a few cases had broken out in Upper Egypt and in the outlying provinces.

John Weir, the Rockefeller Foundation advisor to the Ministry of Health, agreed with Kamal that the early isolation of contacts and cases had contributed much more to the containment of the epidemic than had the vaccination program.[102] Bruce Wilson observed that no one earning more than six pounds a month had contracted the disease.[103] A reasonable standard of living had proven the best protection against cholera.

A. Kordi, a bacteriologist, studied patients in the Abbasiyya Fever Hospital. He found that 24.55 percent of those who had contracted the disease and had not been vaccinated perished from cholera. Of those vaccinated with one dose, 9.81 percent perished; and of those vaccinated with two doses, 8.1 percent perished.[104] These percentages would seem to suggest the efficacy of the vaccination program. But those able to procure two injections may have had better access to potable water, better access to facilities for cooking food and for personal hygiene, and if they were stricken, better access to medical assistance than those who had not been injected or those who had received only one injection.

Cholera patients treated in the Abbasiyya Fever Hospital were greatly aided by new methods of determining the specific gravity of blood. During the epidemic the NAMRU-3 staff learned to measure the specific gravity of the patient's bodily fluid to determine the exact volume and composition of rehydration fluids needed. With this technique, no antibiotics were needed. In one study of forty severely ill patients treated by this method, only three died. While the overall case fatality rate of those treated in isolation centers and elsewhere was 50 percent, the case fatality rate for the three thousand patients treated at Abbasiyya Fever Hospital was 5 percent to 7.5 percent, probably the lowest rate ever achieved to that date.[105]

The British embassy's "General Political Review of 1947" considered the Nuqrashi government's response to the epidemic a notable exception in a year of inaction and apathy.[106] Pridie reported that the government had made "almost superhuman efforts" to control cholera. Although conditions were favorable for the rapid spread of the disease, he said that the doctors had succeeded in checking it and had averted a national calamity.[107] Abd al-Rahman al-Raf'i, the noted nationalistic historian of modern Egypt, agreed with Pridie's assessment. He wrote that the government had launched a valiant campaign against cholera and that the various social classes of Egypt had united in complete solidarity against the epidemic.[108] Al-Raf'i did not, however, mention the troublesome question that had arisen at the beginning of the epidemic. Where had cholera come from?

8

The British Connection

In September 1947 cholera was making news in only one place in the world: the Punjab region of India. British colonial India had just become independent, and the new state of Pakistan was being formed from the western provinces of the former colony. Muslim and Hindu refugees were fleeing horrendous communal strife. On 8 September 1947 cholera had broken out among refugees crossing the Punjab into Pakistan and India. Thousands of British troops being evacuated from India stopped over at Tal al-Kabir base en route to Britain.[1] Tal al-Kabir, where the British had defeated the Egyptian army in 1882, was an ordnance depot and the largest British base outside of India. Although the 1936 Treaty allowed only ten thousand British troops to be stationed in Egypt in peacetime, many times that number were at the base.[2] The possibility that the troops had carried cholera to Egypt seemed entirely plausible.

The possibility of a British connection enraged Egyptian nationalists. Only two days before the outbreak, Prime Minister Nuqrashi had returned from New York where he had presented to the Security Council of the United Nations Egypt's desire to unify with Sudan. To his great disappointment, the council had merely called for negotiations between Britain and Egypt over the future of Sudan. Egyptian nationalists jumped at the chance to use the cholera epidemic to build their case against the British and to strengthen their demand that the British not only evacuate all troops from Egyptian territory but pay reparations to Egypt.

Muhammad Hasanayn Haykal, later the influential editor of *al-Ahram* and close associate of Gamal Abd al-Nasser, atempted to demonstrate that British troops had brought cholera into Egypt. Haykal was at the time a junior reporter for *Akhbar al-Yawm*, which sent him to investigate the outbreak. He subsequently won the King Faruq Prize for Journalism for his articles.[3] In al-Qurayn, Haykal learned that the first two victims, Hasan Khayr Allah and his son, Ragab Hasan Khayr Allah, had worked in the same workshop at the base. The two lived apart in al-Qurayn, and no one else in their households became ill. Another early victim was a foreman in charge of DDT spraying for the British army. Most of the early cases were from al-Bahiriyya in the northern section of al-Qurayn, the section closest to the British base. Al-Qibliyya, the southern section of the town, was farthest from the base and was initially free of the disease. The presumption was that the first victims had contracted the disease at the base. In detective style, Haykal carefully laid out the case against the British. He said that, while the whole story was not yet known, the following facts could be established:

1. Cholera existed in epidemic form only in India.

2. British troops had been moving from India to Egypt.

3. British army authorities said they were surveying their troops for quarantinable diseases.

4. Cholera had broken out in al-Qurayn near the British base.

5. Egyptian workers from al-Qurayn had been in contact with the soldiers.

6. The infection might have come from a cholera carrier who had not developed symptoms of the disease.

7. The Egyptian Quarantine Administration had been carefully surveying all ports for quarantinable diseases.

In addition a "reliable source" informed Haykal that he had been walking with a friend, a British officer, near the hospital at the base when a soldier told the officer to keep away from the isolation area because of the many cases of fever there. He reasoned that there may have been cholera cases among them but admitted that the British categorically denied it.

He then listed three incidents between Egyptian and British troops that led to suspicion regarding the source. In the first incident, on 23 September, two British soldiers tried to pass near the canal despite Egyptian orders forbidding it. The British command apologized and gave assurances that it would not happen again. In the second incident, a car carrying several doctors from the base to the British embassy in Cairo did not arrive on time. A second car went to look for it and passed illegally through the cordon. In the third incident, a British officer claimed his jeep was stolen and went to look for it in the restricted area. The British soldiers had therefore repeatedly ignored Egyptian quarantine restrictions and could have transmitted the disease.

Haykal had interviewed Ministry of Health authorities who told him that they preferred not to dwell on the question of the source but rather to concentrate on combating the epidemic. They would investigate the source when it was under control. Nevertheless, Haykal concluded that cholera must have been imported by British soldiers coming from India.[4]

The allegations against the British reached a crescendo. Publications of all political tendencies shared in the conviction that the British troops were responsible for the epidemic, but the propalace publications, being better funded than the opposition ones, ran the most colorful political cartoons and cover illustrations, condemning the British and linking cholera to wider issues (figs. 20–23). In an unsigned editorial entitled "Political Cholera," *Akhbar al-Yawm* stated that, if the cholera microbe entered via British planes, the political microbe had entered via Britain too. The British hoped to oust Nuqrashi, who had taken Egypt's case to the United Nations, where he had demanded the evacuation of British troops and unity with Sudan. British interests had distorted the economy and caused inflation and inequities. Police and workers at major industries were on strike for higher wages. Both cholera and strikes, the editorial observed, were costing millions of pounds and emptying the treasury.[5]

A fortnight later *Akhbar al-Yawm* suggested that cholera epidemic had occurred because the gap between the rich and the poor was one of the largest in the world and that the extravagance of the elite was unparalleled. It said that Egypt needed social reform, progressive taxation, and an inheritance tax. The government was, according to the article, so far to the right that it would have to move way to the left

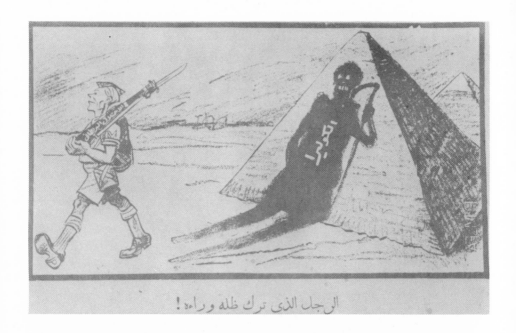

الرجل الذى ترك ظله وراءه !

Fig. 20. "The man who left his shadow behind him." The rifle reads: "British occupation," and the shadow is the specter of death named Cholera." Source: *Akbar al-Yawm,* 4 October 1947.

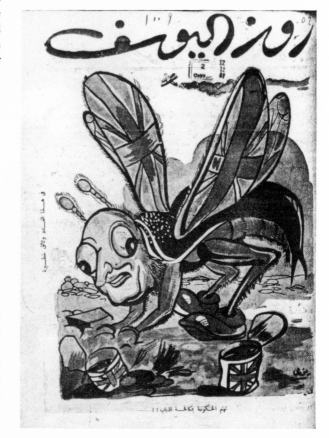

Fig. 21. A British fly (a caricature of Mustafa Nahhas) rooting in a British army dump, with airplanes flying overhead spraying insecticide. The caption reads: "The government is spraying for flies rather than dealing with the real source." Source: *Ruz al-Yusuf,* 1 October 1947.

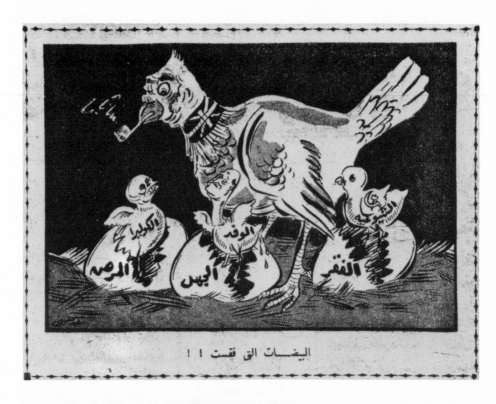

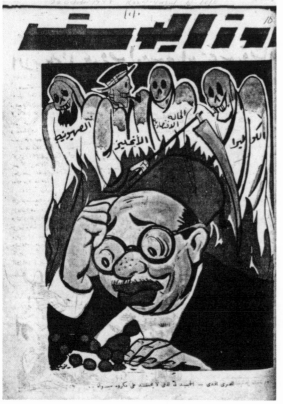

Fig. 22. A British chicken has laid three eggs. Reading right to left the first egg, labeled "Poberty," hatches "Communism"; the second, labeled "Ignorance," hatches the "Wafd"; and the third, labeled "Disease," hatches "Cholera." Source: *Ruz al-Yusuf,* 14 October 1947.

Fig. 23. Masri Effendi beset with four evil spirits: cholera, the economic situation, the British, and Zionism. He comments "Praise God who does not extol such hateful things." Source: *Ruz al-Yusuf,* 22 October 1947.

just to reach the center.[6] Throughout the 1940s the propalace journals had criticized the wealthy elite and had called for social reforms, but the calls remained in the media and were more for propaganda than for action.

The Wafd papers implicated the British as did the others but muted their criticisms. *Al-Misri* wrote that since the five British airfields near Ismailia and the Suez Canal were not subject to Egyptian quarantine, cholera could have been transported by air and not by land or sea, but the newspaper acknowledged that British authorities had finally agreed to let Egyptian quarantine officials supervise the area.[7] *Al-Balagh* ran an article entitled "Lessons We Learn from the Appearance of Cholera." It said that only backward countries could rival Egypt in number of flies.[8] The implication was that Egypt needed to develop its economy to withstand such diseases. The newspaper later stated that since Egyptian doctors had no proof of a British role in transmitting the disease and since the British denied it, the matter should be dropped.[9]

The Muslim Brotherhood went a step further than the other political tendencies, insisting that the British had intentionally brought cholera into Egypt. *Ikhwan al-Muslimin,* the Muslim Brotherhood's weekly journal, charged the British with deliberately using cholera as a weapon to divert Egyptians so that they could detach Sudan from Egypt and add it to the British crown.[10] The daily newspaper of the Muslim Brotherhood, also named *Ikhwan al-Muslimin,* published an "official British military document" dated 11 September 1947 announcing that all filtration plants would increase chlorine dosage to 2.0 parts per million to disinfect the water and stated that a similar order had been issued earlier, on 28 August 1947. This, the newspaper believed, indicated that the British knew of cholera cases sometime before the first cases were discovered in al-Qurayn. The newspaper charged the Nuqrashi government with failure to fight the despicable methods used by the British against the Egyptian people. It concluded that Egyptians knew the true source of the contagion, from which they could be immunized by proper conduct and manly behavior.[11] A few days later the newspaper cited an article in an unnamed morning newspaper in which a high-ranking Ministry of Health official said cholera had come in a British tanker. In addition, the newspaper had found an "official document" issued by British military authorities. The document said that on

28 August 1947 there were three hundred cases of cholera at the British base and that thirty had died per day. The paper charged that the British authorities had not reported the outbreak to the Egyptian authorities and that the Muslim Brotherhood should look into the matter.[12] This last claim of three hundred cases of cholera at the British base is unsubstantiated by other sources and was presumably a fabrication. The Muslim Brotherhood's weekly observed that the route of infection followed the Ismailia canal and that the road running alongside the canal, Treaty Road, symbolized the British connection.[13] The Muslim Brotherhood claimed that the only solution for the cholera epidemic was a *jihad* (holy war) against imperialism. *Jihad* alone would result in liberty and independence. The British were the root of the epidemic because they drained the country of resources. Cholera was like an invading army and the government was right to fight it, but the real enemies were foreign occupation and colonization. The *umma* (Egyptian people) would eventually win independence and establish an Islamic society.[14] Since the three enemies, poverty, disease, and ignorance, had not killed the people and destroyed the nation, the British, according to the Muslim Brotherhood, had brought the microbe to depopulate Egypt and to divert people from the cause of nationalism. The British sent an outdated cholera vaccine to poison the people, but the Ministry of Health had forbidden its use.[15] There is no corroborating evidence to support any of these claims.

The Muslim Brotherhood praised the king, who had asked in the Chamber of Deputies if the government was in fact fighting poverty, disease, and ignorance and had criticized it for concentrating its efforts on model villages that diverted genuine social reform.[16] In 1947 the Muslim Brotherhood had allied with the palace in an effort to outmaneuver the Wafd party.

Minbar al-Sharq, a monthly magazine published by the Muslim Brotherhood, wrote that the epidemic was both an affliction and a blessing. It was an affliction for the stricken but a blessing for the government because they could conceal their actions from the distracted public.[17] Abd al-Aziz al-Zuhayri, a well-known member of the Muslim Brotherhood, wrote that the only way to deal with cholera was to return to Islamic law and morality: God developed the microbe and kept it away from those He wished to spare. Fourteen centuries ago God warned people to repent and atone for their wrongdoings. The true reason for the epidemic was the obscenity in Egypt: "God is angry with us and is punishing us for the bars and for the advertisements of liquor seen in newspapers and on billboards. We must prevent usury, which God forbids and Egypt allows. We must prevent girls from being immoral. Once immoral girls and liquor advertisements disappear from the streets and the press, the malaise will disappear. Vaccine is of no use; another epidemic will come. Everything is from God."[18]

The Muslim Brotherhood therefore supported the palace, blamed the British troops, and linked Egypt's social problems to colonization. They also believed that the cholera outbreak illustrated the need for a *jihad* against both imperialism and immorality and for the establishment of a new society based on Islamic law.

Al-Jamahir, published by Haditu, the communist coalition party, blamed British troops for bringing the disease and declared that cholera was a political disease, an epidemic of colonies existing only in places like China and India, where the forces of imperialism had resulted in poverty and illiteracy. The government had said people should go back to work or to school, but how could they when colonization was hindering the economic revolution of the country? Students and workers should be receiving military training to fight the imperialist forces, which now included not only Britain but the United States.[19] The following week, *al-Jamahir* reported that everything was collapsing. The country was being paralyzed by cholera and by large-scale strikes of judges, engineers, government employees, and workers in the Shell Oil Company at Suez and in the national textile industries. The wave of strikes was like an epidemic. Both were rooted in colonization, which siphoned profits from the workers' salaries. The Nuqrashi government, the newspaper charged, was subservient to foreign companies. Vaccine was not the cure for the epidemic: the only cure was the evacuation of British troops and improvement in the standard of living.[20]

Khalid Muhammad Khalid, the progressive Islamic *alim* (religious scholar) who advocated socialism under Islamic law, wrote an article in *al-Jamahir* in which he criticized a Friday *khutbah* on cholera prepared and distributed to the mosques by the Ministry of Waqfs. He observed that the cholera *khutbah* discussed everything but the real reason for cholera, which was poverty. Poverty had already led to malaria among the people of Upper Egypt, and now once again poverty paved the way for the current battle of death.[21] *Al-Jamahir* thus blamed the cholera epidemic and all of Egypt's ills on British imperialism, which blocked the economic revolution that would eliminate poverty. The logical solution was to work to eliminate British imperialism and, with aid from the Soviet Union, to establish a socialist society.[22]

Ahmad Husayn, founder of Young Egypt, took a different tack. He said that, while the British had caused the epidemic by turning their base into a state within a state, preventing surveillance by the Egyptian Quarantine Administration, it should not be allowed to divert people from the real cause, which was total independence from Britain. Any nation, he reasoned, could experience a natural disaster. Husayn called on the government to resign because it had not solved Egypt's many problems and called on the fellahin to revolt against the palace.[23] He observed that losses from cholera were few in comparison with the 1942–44 malaria epidemic in Qina and Aswan in which one hundred thousand persons had died. Cholera could, however, be dealt with through modern medical advances, which had not been available in 1902 when the last epidemic had ravaged Egypt. Like the other opposition parties, he complained that government statistics for cholera deaths were not accurate, that people were forced into isolation camps, which lacked adequate provisions, but that the real problems facing Egypt remained evacuation of British troops and unity of the Nile Valley. If Young Egypt were to come to power, Ahmad Husayn vowed that all landlords would be compelled to live among their fellahin.[24]

The British embassy repeatedly denied the accusations that British troops were responsible for the outbreak. On 25 September the British embassy had announced in the *Egyptian Gazette* that, while no cases had appeared among British troops in Egypt, cases had appeared among Egyptians working in Ismailia and the Suez Canal. The implication was that cholera had been transmitted by passengers traveling by ship through the canal. The newspaper noted that the Muslim Brotherhood had preserved their traditional line of blaming the British for everything. This time it was the cholera epidemic.[25] In response to further accusations, the embassy published a notice in the *Egyptian Gazette* stating that British vaccines were pure and effective.[26] The embassy reported to London that "there had been further malicious allegations that the outbreak is attributable to the presence of British forces in Egypt and suitable material has been published by this embassy to refute this charge. The Ministry of Health has categorically rebutted an allegation in the Moslem Brethren's newspaper that serum sent from the United Kingdom was stale and useless."[27] The newspaper highlighted a rather improbable story taken from *Sawt al-Umma,* a satirical journal published by the left wing of the Wafd party, which had claimed that a test tube containing cholera microbes had been stolen from the ministry's laboratories four months before. Could the flask, the journal asked, have been the source of the epidemic?[28] This possibility seems to have been sensibly ignored by the rest of the Arabic press.

The accusations against the British took a new turn on 26 October 1947, when Huda Sha'rawi, president of the Egyptian Feminist Union, sent a statement to the United Nations accusing the British of having brought the epidemic to Egypt.[29] She began by stating that despite denials issued by the British embassy in Cairo and official quarters in London, the Egyptian Feminist Union held the British occupation forces responsible for the outbreak and spread of cholera in Egypt. She cited as evidence that the first cases had broken out in al-Qurayn among workers employed on the Tal al-Kabir base. Furthermore, British military authorities had not only evaded all control and ignored international quarantine regulations but had dismissed the Egyptian workers without first notifying the local authorities that they should undertake the necessary cholera-control measures. In the name of the Egyptian Feminist Union, she appealed to the United Nations and to world opinion to help Egypt free itself from the British occupation.[30]

Apparently the United Nations took no action on this statement. The House of Commons did take it up, and Henry Morris-Jones, a member of Parliament, asked Ernest Bevin, the secretary of state for foreign affairs, to clarify the matter. Morris-Jones wanted to know what measures had been taken to mitigate the effect of such propaganda on British relations with Egypt and other countries. Bevin replied that the "extreme attack" was unworthy of a reply and would only be believed by those already hopelessly prejudiced against the British. Morris-Jones asked if Bevin was aware that he could not "dismiss the matter so peremptorily as all that? This lady is not an irresponsible person in Egypt, and surely we cannot allow these statements to pass without taking steps to contradict them."[31] Bevin said that he had announced the previous week everything that the British government had done for Egypt and had been thanked in person by the Egyptian ambassador in London. Asked whether assistance would continue, Bevin said that he had just learned that John Taylor and Bruce White, both noted British cholera experts, were in Egypt to carry out research on cholera and would be available to assist the Egyptian authorities.[32]

The British War Office subsequently issued an official communiqué announcing again that there had been no cases of cholera among the British troops in Egypt, which, it said, was due to preventive measures taken by the British military authorities. There were, however, two cases among the African troops under British command: both men had recovered. Despite reports to the contrary, the two cases had occurred after the outbreak among the Egyptian population, not before. The communiqué concluded that senior officers ascribed the immunity of British troops to their own discipline and good sense.[33] The embassy issued a second communiqué on 10 November stating that the claim published by *Akhbar al-Yawm*, that British civilians had been immunized against cholera before it appeared on 20 September, was "completely untrue."[34]

The Lancet, Britain's leading medical journal, covered the epidemic extensively. The first article on the outbreak suggested that pilgrims returning from Mecca may have brought the disease back to Egypt.[35] In response, an Egyptian doctor residing in Switzerland sent a letter to the editor of *The Lancet* noting that Mecca was, because of the efficient quarantining of pilgrims, no longer a center of disease spread. However, he said that British troops had carried malaria and relapsing fever to Egypt during the last war and could have introduced cholera now.[36] The editor replied that all of the charges were groundless and that there was no evidence that the *Anopheles gambiae* mosquito was carried into Egypt by British troops by land, air, or water. Relapsing fever had, he said, been nearly nonexistent among British troops during the war but was epidemic in Egypt from time to time. Finally, the suggestion that cholera was introduced into Egypt by troop movements from India broke down in the face of there having been no cases of cholera among British troops in India, among those stationed or arriving in the Canal Zone, or among the peoples of the Middle East as a whole.[37]

In the next issue the editor stated that al-Qurayn was near the Canal Zone, which suggested that a ship might have carried an undetected case aboard, or a commercial airplane in Lower Egypt might have carried an undetected case.[38] This article was republished in the *Egyptian Gazette*.[39]

The following week *The Lancet* published another article, this time suggesting that the epidemic was in fact brought in by British troops. The article, by "a correspondent in Egypt," repeated the by now familiar opinion that, while the source of the epidemic remained obscure and no official statement concerning its source had been made, many firsthand observers believed it could be traced to Egyptians who worked in British army airports not under the supervision of the Egyptian Quarantine Administration. The correspondent repeated the observation that cholera had broken out in the Punjab in August and that British airmen returning from India used the base as a quarantine station, remaining there with their Indian retainers for two weeks before departing for England. Furthermore the correspondent noted that there was no connection between the epidemic and the pilgrimage.[40] *The Lancet* had thus hedged its bets and offered both sides of the argument to its readers. This second article was *not* republished in the *Egyptian Gazette*.

Egyptian medical experts sharply disagreed about the question of the source of the cholera. Khalil Abd al-Khaliq angrily insisted that the British had brought in the disease. He had reason to be angry: he had just been dismissed from his post as undersecretary of health for the Quarantine Administration.

Antagonisms had been building for some time. In April 1947 he had read a paper before the Royal Egyptian Medical Association in which he repeated the charges that the British were responsible for both the malaria and the relapsing fever epidemics. He had insisted that Egypt had suffered more war-related casualties than the United States, that Egypt should be compensated for its sacrifices during the war, and that the 1936 Treaty endangered Egypt and should be abolished.[41] In an international health conference in Paris in April and May 1946, he had recommended that passengers departing from cholera-infected areas be detained for five days at the port of departure, where they could be examined by physicians. France, Britain, India, and other nations had opposed the motion because it was impractical to detain so many people, and it did not carry, he bitterly recalled. He said the nations of the world laughed at Egypt for being too lax but criticized it when it urged extra vigilance.[42]

On 11 March and 1 May 1947, when British troops were being withdrawn to the Suez Canal, Abd al-Khaliq had sent two letters to Nuqrashi, advising closer Egyptian quarantine surveillance of British troops. Nuqrashi, however, took the position that Egypt had no right to survey British military airports or bases until the 1936 Treaty was renegotiated.[43]

The plot had thickened when Abd al-Khaliq persuaded the Ministry of Health to issue a decree forming a Pan-Arab Health Bureau, with Egypt as its first member. Membership would be based on a national and ethnic basis rather than on a geographic basis. Meanwhile, Ali Tawfiq Shusha had begun negotiations for Egyptian participation in another international health organization associated with the United Nations to be called the World Health Organization.

An earlier and similar health unit had been formed as a branch of the League of Nations following World War I. When the League of Nations had collapsed, its health section had disbanded. In consequence the United Nations agreed to the formation of a separate public health organization with its headquarters in Geneva rather than in New York. Plans for the organization were made in 1945 and 1946, when the Interim Commission was formed. The commission oversaw the drawing up and ratification of the organization's constitution, the establishment and coordination of regional organizations, and the daily working of the organization until it was formally convened. According to the philosophy of the new organization, human beings had a right to more than mere freedom from disease. They also had a right to physical and mental well-being, and it was the obligation of governments to ensure this. Since the health of all peoples was essential for world peace and for political stability, it was justified in being a major concern of the United Nations.[44]

Shusha, a strong supporter of the World Health Organization, considered Abd al-Khaliq obstructive in his efforts to establish the Pan-Arab Health Bureau. The British embassy agreed. Pridie, the health counselor to the British embassy, reported in May 1947 that all British officials who had had dealings with Abd al-Khaliq during and after the war had distrusted him and found him extremely politically minded and violently anti-British.[45] The embassy urged that Egypt, Sudan, and the other Arab states in which it had influence not join the Pan-Arab Health Bureau until the World Health Organization had decided on its own format. Then they would join the regional division of the World Health Organization, not the Pan-Arab Health Bureau, thus preventing a fait accompli.[46]

On 25 May 1947 Nuqrashi transferred Abd al-Khaliq from the Quarantine Administration to a research position, replacing him with Muhammad Nazif, who, according to the British Foreign Office, was likely to have views different from his predecessor.[47] Nazif promptly flew to Geneva, where he negotiated Egypt's membership in the World Health Organization. Alexandria became its regional headquarters, and Shusha became Egypt's first representative.

Abd al-Khaliq spent his time during the epidemic insisting that his policies, if they had been carried out, would have averted the outbreak. He wrote the Minister of Health to remind him of his urgent request that all arrivals from India be bacteriologically examined to discover any possible cholera carriers and that this had not been done.[48] He charged that an engineer among the troops coming from India had died of cholera before 23 September 1947, the beginning of the cholera outbreak.[49] He did not reveal his source for this unsubstantiated piece of information.

He criticized the Ministry of Health for having permitted two World Health Organization experts, W. W. Yung and P. M. Kaul, to investigate the source of the epidemic because they were from a foreign agency. Locating the source was, he said, an internal Egyptian affair. He claimed that the two experts had ruled out the British connection on the grounds that the outbreak had begun simultaneously in three villages, not all of which contributed laborers to the British bases, and that they had suggested that a ship in the Suez canal or overland travelers from China, Malaya, or French Indochina may have brought the disease into Egypt.[50] Despite Abd al-Khaliq's impassioned claims, the World Health Organization did not conclude that cholera had been brought into Egypt by overland travelers (as will be seen below).

Abd al-Khaliq wrote numerous articles vociferously attacking the

British. He reasoned that because cholera was officially reported in the Punjab in the week of 31 August to 6 September, British planes probably transferred cholera carriers during the second week of September. Cases must have appeared at the British base about 11 September 1947 because on that day general headquarters issued an order to increase the amount of chlorine in the base's drinking water. The British, he said, did not deny the existence of the order.[51] This was, however, guilt by very tenuous association.

Dr. Sa'id Abduh, assistant professor of hygiene and preventive medicine at Fuad I University, shared Khalil Abd al-Khaliq's attitudes. Abduh wrote extensively about the epidemic in newspapers and in scholarly journals. He said he had received a letter from an unnamed Egyptian doctor saying that British subjects had received an order to go to Cairo the first week of September to get a cholera vaccination. This might, he reasoned, be expected in a country like India, where cholera was endemic, but not in Egypt, where there had been no cholera for forty-five years. The same doctor mentioned that British engineers at Kafr al-Dawwar, a town in Lower Egypt, were not at work on 6 September 1947. When asked why, they replied that they were on strike, but in fact they were in Cairo getting vaccinations against cholera.[52] Abduh's allegation is not substantiated by other sources.

Shusha took a much more cautious approach to the matter. The respected newspaper *al-Ahram* interviewed him in early October and asked him what he thought about the repeated claims that the epidemic had been introduced from the British base. Shusha replied that high-ranking doctors in the British army often came to his office to discuss the medical problems of Egyptian workers. He had asked them if they had noticed any suspected cases of cholera among their troops, and they had denied it completely.[53] He later published an article on the 1947 cholera epidemic in the first edition of the *Bulletin of the World Health Organization* but avoided the question of the epidemic's source.[54]

Nazif, Abd al-Khaliq's replacement as undersecretary of health for the Quarantine Administration, also avoided the issue. At the meeting of the World Health Organization in Geneva, called to discuss the epidemic, he merely described the outbreak and invited opinions about its source.[55] The Ministry of Health officials preferred to distance themselves from the explosive political question.

In November 1947, the Ministry of Health had finally appointed a committee of experts to study the source of the epidemic. Abd al-Khaliq and Sa'id Abduh soon criticized the committee for taking too much time. Muhammad Nazif rebuked them and said neither knew anything about the workings of the committee or of the extensive study undertaken by Ministry of Health experts to find the answer.[56] At the end of December, *al-Assas,* the ruling Sa'dist party's newspaper, sent a journalist to ask Nagib Iskandar, the minister of health, what the committee had found. Iskandar said that the committee had begun its work by delineating the region in which cholera had appeared. The British authorities had been on guard against such an epidemic coming by sea or air via military transport. Iskandar said that he hoped to conclude the study decisively, so that the question would not come up again.[57] In its annual report the Ministry of Health gave only a few lines to the cholera epidemic and said that the special committee that had been convened would submit a complete report.[58] The complete report was never published.

A. M. Kamal, the director of preventive medicine for the Ministry of Health and one of Egypt's pioneers in the field of epidemiology, never published his views on the question of source.[59] According to his son-in-law Salah Atiyya, a noted physician and World Health Organization consultant, Kamal did not attribute the epidemic to the British. He thought there were other unverifiable sources of contact. Date traders and smugglers of military goods, for example, had long established themselves in al-Qurayn. Bedouin traveling to and from Egypt across the Sinai were not subject to quarantine checks. No cases of cholera had broken out among the Bedouin, however, nor were there any cases in Palestine. Kamal concluded only that cholera "came from outside Egypt."[60]

Bruce Wilson and John Weir suspected that the first cases had actually appeared near al-Qurayn at the village of Kafr Hamza about two weeks before the outbreak was announced. Two sisters had died there of a disease diagnosed as food poisoning. On 10 September there were about ten deaths in and around Kafr Hamza.[61] Kafr Hamza was farther away from the Tal al-Kabir base than was al-Qurayn and therefore had fewer contacts with it, which might have helped exonerate the British, but their suspicions were not confirmed.

In mid-December, Fuad Sirag al-Din, in a Senate interpellation, accused the British of having imported the disease and the Nuqrashi government of negligence in not having taken extra precautions when cholera had broken out in India in late August. He claimed that the government had undermined the quarantine service by transferring Khalil Abd al-Khaliq and added that the disease would not have entered Egypt if Abd al-Khaliq's recommendations of April and May 1946 had been carried out.[62] He regretted that the ministry had not heeded Abd al-Khaliq's advice during the epidemic; he also regretted that Nazif had told the World Health Organization that the disease had been introduced by overland travelers. He stated that the government was not interested in finding the source because it was a "political source." All the world knew the source; the minister of health knew the source but did not want to say it.[63] Iskandar replied that there was no way to be certain the disease had come by air just because the ports were surveyed by quarantine officials. Many epidemics, he said, had entered through surveyed ports.[64] Nazif had only mentioned the possibility that travelers from other infected countries may have been the source. He said that Abd al-Khaliq had sent to him seventy-seven reports of at least ten pages each to keep him from doing his work during the epidemic.[65]

The following day Sirag al-Din repeated the criticisms against the government. Iskandar and Shusha defended the government's actions, promised that the committee that had been set up to study the source of the epidemic would soon issue a final report, and thanked the international donors and the benevolent societies for their help. After several hours of discussion, the interpellation ended with the senators voting to thank the government.[66]

Nur al-Din Tarraf, a member of Hizb al-Watani (the National party) and a prominent physician and professor of medicine at Ayn Shams University, then made an interpellation in the Chamber of Deputies.[67] He insisted that the 1936 Treaty did not grant special privileges to the British to disregard Egyptian quarantine procedures except during wartime. During the war, therefore, plague had entered through the Suez Canal; malaria through Wadi Halfa, Sudan; and relapsing fever through the western desert. After the war British pilots had continued to refuse to follow Egyptian quarantine regulations, resulting in the cholera epidemic. He claimed that John Taylor, the British cholera expert, had confirmed that cholera was carried by airplane into Egypt from India.[68]

Iskandar replied that the British had not violated Egyptian quarantine regulations because there was no agreement concerning military aircraft landing at Fayid Airport in the Canal Zone. He said the government should be credited with having successfully carried out the first mass vaccination in the history of cholera epidemics. With that the Chamber of Deputies voted to thank the government, and the interpellation—but not the controversy—ended.

P. M. Kaul, one of the two World Health Organization cholera experts who had visited Egypt during the cholera epidemic, and Yves Biraud, the organization's director of epidemiology and public health statistics, prepared the final report for the World Health Organization. The report concluded that, while all of the six epidemics in Egypt in the previous century—those in 1830, 1848, 1865, 1883, 1895, and 1902—had originated in the Mecca pilgrimages, where cholera had been introduced by Indian pilgrims, the 1947 epidemic had broken out nearly one month before the return of the pilgrims. Furthermore cholera had not appeared in Mecca or Medina since 1914. Biraud and Kaul concluded that the Egyptian authorities believed that the infection had been brought over from India, and they quoted from *Lancet*'s article by the unnamed correspondent, suggesting that British troops had imported it.[69] The World Health Organization therefore neither confirmed nor denied the allegations that the British army was responsible for the cholera epidemic.

By early December the British agreed to an investigation of the Tal al-Kabir base by high-ranking British researchers in collaboration with Egyptian medical experts. All parties agreed that the investigation would be carried out on a "purely scientific basis."[70] Records of this investigation should be found in the Public Record Office in London. The *Foreign Office Index* lists numerous documents under the heading: "1947: Diseases: Cholera: Epidemic in Egypt." For example, one file is entitled "Egyptian Allegations and Propaganda Regarding British Medical Assistance and Responsibility for Epidemic: Report of Investigations by British Officials: F.O. Comments: P.Qs." A second file is entitled "Investigation into Origin of: F.O. Proposals Regarding Setting of Board of Inquiry." Documents pertaining to the epidemic were still appearing in the *Foreign Office Index* of 1949. One file is entitled "Egyptian Epidemic: Conclusions as to Origin."[71] None of these records can be found today.

Public Record Office librarians explain that, although records from the 1940s have been opened to the public under the thirty-year rule, many documents have been destroyed for reasons of space. From mid-1946 until the early 1950s, many, but not all, items relating to medicine and disease in Egypt have apparently been destroyed. All the malaria and relapsing fever records are, however, in place. The British Ministry of Health, the Egyptian Ministry of Health, the London School of Tropical Medicine and Hygiene, and the National Research Institute at Mill Hill, London, have no copies of any of the items mentioned above.

Opinions remained divided about the source of the epidemic. In 1950 Egypt's representative to the World Health Organization reproached representatives from Britain, India, and Pakistan for negligence in applying quarantine regulations in 1947.[72] The *British Medical Journal* stated in 1951 that the source of infection remained a mystery and that cholera had struck throughout the Canal Zone—except among British troops.[73] Medical administrators at the al-Qurayn hospital whom I interviewed in 1985 believe that Indian Muslims who were attached to the British air force used to come to al-Qurayn to pray because the base did not have a mosque and that cholera carriers may have transmitted the disease while performing ablutions before prayer. Ministry of Health officials I interviewed in Cairo in 1986 suggest that people scavenging in the garbage dump outside the base may have contracted the disease from contaminated refuse.

If the missing records ever surface, they may indicate the presence of a cholera carrier among the troops or among the Indian workers at the base, or there may be no records of such a cholera carrier. That all of the records are missing may, of course, suggest a cover-up.

Although the source of the epidemic was never decisively proven and reparations were never paid, the public was convinced the British troops had brought it to Egypt. Many people came to share the view of Taha Husayn (1889–1973), one of the foremost Egyptian writers of the twentieth century. In September 1947 Husayn had been returning to Egypt by ship from France when he heard the first news of the epidemic. He had lost his older brother to cholera in the 1902 epidemic and was horrified at the news. Back in Cairo, in the midst of the epidemic, he wrote that catastrophes were coming from every direction. Though Egypt had built schools, a Ministry of Health, and modern institutions of government since the 1902 epidemic, its people were still victims of poverty, illiteracy, and disease, and their leaders were still dominated by their British masters. Britain had valued Egypt's support during the war, but once the war had been won, the British conspired against the Egyptian people. Egypt was, Taha Husayn said, blessed with a fertile land and a clear sky, which should have resulted in better living conditions.[74] The British connection seemed to manifest Egypt's victimization by outside forces. Cholera had become a metaphor for all that was wrong with Egypt.

9

Public Health on the
National Agenda

Following the cholera epidemic, talk of public-health reform was in the air. The Egyptian government vowed to increase potable water supplies, to open several new hospitals and rural health units, and to introduce a progressive taxation law that was designed to alleviate the poverty that had been so dramatically associated with the epidemic. The Minister of Health lamented, "We have about 4,500 doctors in Egypt, of whom 1,400 are in government service. If we had 1,200 more, we would have an average of one doctor per 5,000 inhabitants. We have 21,000 hospital beds, one for 800 inhabitants, where in England the average is one for every ten persons."[1] Habib Ayrout, after quoting this comment, notes that of the fourteen hundred doctors only six hundred worked in Egypt's four thousand villages, where they were poorly accommodated and poorly paid.[2] To remedy the situation, one medical school had been established at Faruq University in Alexandria in 1942, a second at Dimirdash Hospital in Cairo in 1945, and a third was to be established at Tanta in 1950.[3] The newer schools were, however, inadequately equipped and staffed.

Egypt's political leaders renewed their promises to improve the government's public-health and medical services. It was, however, an era of increasing political instability and uncertainty: on 28 December 1948 the Muslim Brotherhood organization assassinated Prime Minister Nuqrashi, who had recently prohibited its activities. The government promptly closed all of the brotherhood's political and medical facilities and confiscated all of their equipment, educational materials, and party literature.⁴ On 12 February 1949 government agents assassinated Hasan al-Banna, founder of the Muslim Brotherhood. The government, now led by Ibrahim Abd al-Hadi, a former minister of health and deputy director of the ruling Sa'dist party, incarcerated thousands of communists, Zionists, brotherhood members, and other dissidents in internment camps and banned all political gatherings. The internal-reform programs stalled.

Fikri Abaza, the noted journalist and political critic, wrote in *al-Musawwar* that Egyptians had once blamed all of their problems on the British occupation. Then other excuses were found, such as the government's inexperience, the difficulties of World War II, and the defeat in the Palestine War. For years, he said, people had spoken of reforming the taxation system and of extending irrigation and facilities for potable water, but the reforms always became bogged down in the machinery of government. Now was the time to stop blaming outsiders and to take action.⁵ *Akhir Sa'a* published an unsigned editorial, which stated that the masses had no confidence or trust in the upper classes because Egypt's leaders had paid more attention to attacking one another than to carrying out social programs, a practice that had led to instability, to a breakdown in morality, to anarchy, and to extremist ideologies that flourished in a terrain "plowed by despair, deception, fury, hatred, envy, and deprivation."⁶ The editorial praised the success of the Nuqrashi government in dealing with cholera and its promises to raise the standard of living of all the people. Yet, it lamented, the country remained badly in need of reforms to which the rich should contribute.⁷

Ahmad Husayn, president of Young Egypt, announced a new socialist line for his party in 1949. After returning from a four-month visit to Britain, he complained that recent governments had carried out no reforms of any significance. They had only set up a few model villages, factories, clinics, and beggars' rehabilitation centers, which did nothing about the roots of the problem. Young Egypt prepared one hundred thousand copies of a manifesto condemning the government and calling for a new anticommunist, nationalist, and socialist government.⁸

An editorial in *al-Misri,* the Wafdist newspaper, stated that the fellahin were used to hearing promises of reduction of land rents and of projects to improve their standard of living. Then each government, once in power, failed to act on its promises. Even the plan to provide potable water that was begun during the cholera epidemic had fallen apart. The editorial concluded that the time had come for politicians to address the problems of the fellahin who lived in houses not fit for animals, who ate poor-quality bread, who in winter could not buy clothes to protect themselves from the cold, and who drank contaminated water, thus filling their bodies with microbes and worms. The fellahin, despite their misery, worked loyally, planting and cultivating the land to fill the government's coffers and the pockets of the wealthy with gold. Like the other political parties, the Wafd insisted that it alone could carry out the necessary reforms and noted that previous Wafd governments had passed workman's compensation acts and made free education a state responsibility.[9] The editorial was a bit misleading. The workman's compensation acts were limited in scope, and free education was to await Taha Husayn's Ministry of Education in the next Wafdist government. The party had, however, made labor, educational, and public-health reform a central part of its political platform.

Meanwhile the government continued its policy of expanding political influence through emergency relief assistance, this time, in Sudan, which Egypt claimed. In April 1949 the Ministry of Supplies arranged to send £E 50,000 and a Red Crescent mission to famine-stricken regions of Sudan. The British civil secretary of Sudan told the Egyptian government that the situation was well in hand and that the Egyptian aid was not needed.[10] The British were trying to keep the Egyptians from reinforcing their presence in Sudan. Two years earlier, the palace had been somewhat more successful in sending emergency assistance abroad. In April 1947 Faruq had announced that the government would send two military planes carrying twelve army officers, volunteers from the Red Crescent, and 320 tons of wheat to Tunisia and Tripoli to alleviate a famine. The French colonial authorities in Tunisia said that the Tunisians were not starving, that the wheat was not needed, and that the affair had a manifestly political character. The British military authorities in Tripoli, suspecting that Egypt was trying to expand its political influence there and to press its claim to Libyan territory, insisted that the situation was under control and refused to allow Egyptian relief efforts. Then the French and British authorities offered to distribute the relief supplies themselves. Finally after much discussion and delay the French and British authorities had agreed to let the Egyptian missions distribute the wheat.[11] The palace was now accustomed to linking its relief work to its political policies.

Both the British and the American authorities continued to link international assistance, now usually called *bilateral aid,* to their foreign policies. Following the cholera outbreak the British embassy hoped to restore its damaged public image by participating in the public health reforms. Ronald Campbell, the British ambassador, was particularly interested in the project to make potable water available to all the villages of Egypt. Nuqrashi had announced this plan just after the cholera epidemic had ended. When the Egyptian government began taking tenders for extending the existing potable water system, he wrote Bevin that the scheme was "from all points of view, particularly from social and political aspects, the most important development scheme which has been mooted for several years in Egypt."[12] Campbell urged the government to agree to supply materials for the project because it would contribute to the Egyptian government's campaign to improve rural public health and would bring "considerable goodwill" to the British. The Egyptian water purification scheme was, he stated, an enormous undertaking because 13 to 14 million of Egypt's 18 to 19 million people used water taken directly from the Nile, the only source of water in Egypt.[13] The foreign office in London authorized provision of the requested piping and other supplies. British assistance enabled the Egyptian government to supply more than two thousand villages with latrines and potable water. The project was not completed, however, and most of the pumps and water systems broke down within two years because there were no funds for maintenance.[14] The British government wrote off most of the supplies against the debt the British government had owed the Egyptian government since World War II. Some bitterness was caused by the British practice of valuing the British pound equal to the Egyptian pound, though the Egyptian pound was then valued slightly higher in open trading.

According to the British embassy's annual review of 1947, Egypt's preoccupation with foreign affairs had forestalled any serious attempt to improve the miserable conditions in which a majority of its own population lived.[15] The political climate indicated that British authorities should "hasten slowly" to support social reform to ensure that it be along British rather than communist lines. The embassy advocated introducing such reforms by working through influential officials, the women's benevolent societies, and the press.[16]

Britain still worried about American designs on Egypt. In a report to the foreign office on financial and economic conditions in Egypt, the embassy recommended that British experts assist in long-term planning and that Americans not be invited to participate until plans had reached an advanced stage. Since British experts were welcome in the fields of health and education, they should infiltrate only those fields until the political climate changed enough to allow long-term planning. The report concluded that Egyptians were increasingly reluctant to accept foreign advice unless it was "under the counter and on their own terms."[17] The British embassy eventually organized a "Green Crescent" publicity organization, which was in fact only a reading room where Egyptians could find materials on social reform and on British assistance to Egypt.[18] Because of the political climate in both Britain and Egypt, British assistance remained restricted. In the meantime, American public health assistance was increasing.

The Rockefeller Foundation and NAMRU-3 both found that their efforts during the relapsing fever and cholera epidemics had resulted in increased acceptance by the Egyptian public-health establishment. In 1947 John Weir, who had succeeded Bruce Wilson as field staff director of the Africa and Asia Minor Region of the International Health Division of the Rockefeller Foundation, made a survey of Egypt's medical services and public-health services. The purpose of the report was to develop a cooperative program between the Ministry of Health and the Rockefeller Foundation.[19] The report found that the rural health units were treating the very diseases that they should be preventing and that the Ministry of Health, in responding to political pressures, was building more facilities than could be staffed with trained personnel. It recommended the creation of field training centers, the decentralization of local services, the development within the Ministry of Health of a board of trained technical advisers, the establishment of model villages, and a school of public-health nursing. The Rockefeller Foundation offered to provide personnel for the model health unit for at least three to five years.[20]

In response to the recommendations, the Ministry of Health created the Section of Rural Research under the direction of John Weir. The section made a four-year study (1948–52) of the health and sanitation conditions of Egyptian villages. It found that there were 205 rural health units. Each unit was expected to have a doctor, a nurse-midwife, and several assistants serving fifteen thousand to twenty thousand people. The doctor on the average saw ninety new patients per day and attended to numerous other duties, which included prenatal care, bilharzia treatment, sanitary administration, and extensive bureaucratic obligations.[21] The work load was, of course, acute. The study found that government medical services provided about 70 percent of rural medical care. The remaining 30 percent of medical services was obtained through private doctors. Indigenous practitioners were not mentioned, although they probably provided extensive medical services. The Weir study concluded that improvement in health could not be made while the economic and social level of the villagers was such that they must necessarily live in mud-brick houses and keep their farm animals within their homes.[22] It recommended that the government health services be coordinated and that the rural health workers have autonomy of action under village councils.[23] In 1948 the Ministry of Health, with assistance from the Rockefeller Foundation, NAMRU-3, and the World Health Organization, began to develop a model village project at Qalyub in Lower Egypt. But the project was terminated within a few years.

NAMRU-3 managed to obtain its official recognition from the Egyptian government following the cholera epidemic. In mid-February 1948 the Nuqrashi government announced that it had signed an agreement with NAMRU-3 to lease a two-and-one-half-acre plot of land adjacent to the Abbasiyya Fever Hospital to the U.S. government for a twenty-five-year period at a nominal rent.[24] The agreement had to be ratified by Parliament, but its success was nearly assured because in 1948 the Parliament was dominated by the ruling Sa'dist–Liberal Constitutionalist coalition. The agreement symbolized the new American military role in the Mediterranean and in Egypt.

Media response to the agreement suggested that, despite the goodwill NAMRU-3 had won during the cholera epidemic, many Egyptians were opposed to the establishment of an American military facility on Egyptian soil. When the government announced the agreement, opposition newspapers immediately attacked it. The Wafd paper, *al-Misri*, called the establishment of NAMRU-3 proof that the U.S. government was undertaking a "new occupation" near Egyptian military installations.[25] The Egyptian government, the paper said, had surrendered to the armed forces of a foreign government a year after Egypt celebrated the evacuation of British troops from Cairo and that, while NAMRU-3 said that its purpose was only medical research, this claim could not be taken seriously because the world had witnessed many kinds of imperialism in the past that had initially appeared innocent. *Al-Misri* hoped that public opinion, which the government ignored, would force Parliament to reject the new foreign occupation.[26] *Al-Kutla* complained that the Egyptian government would have no control over the new American installation and asked the Nuqrashi government to explain why it would allow a foreign government to carry out military research without surveillance of any kind.[27] Perhaps it was better, the paper said, simply to state that American domination was replacing British domination and that this defeat was due to the subservience of the government to foreign interests. Even the propalace magazine *al-Musawwar* complained that the U.S. Navy had come to Egypt and surveyed restricted and unrestricted areas with advanced equipment. The British embassy had warned the Egyptian Ministry of Foreign Affairs about the American surveillance, but the warning had come too late. The Americans, it concluded, had already left with the results of their inquiries, research, and maps, with no accountability to the Egyptian government.[28] Egypt seemed to be ceding part of its sovereignty to the Americans.

Despite such protests in the media Parliament ratified the plan to lease the land to NAMRU-3, and the final agreement was signed on 28 June 1948.[29] NAMRU-3 was formally dedicated on Navy Day, 27 October 1948. The occasion offered an opportunity to express the widespread postwar view that science and technology could rise above political differences and help the world advance.

In his dedication speech, Commander Phillips briefly described the background and purpose of NAMRU-3. He hoped that the research unit would attract scientists from all over the world who would bring their abilities to Egypt, where they would participate together in the international fight against disease.[30] Nagib Iskandar, the minister of health, said in his address that the research carried out at NAMRU-3 had already been of benefit to epidemiology the world over. In ringing tones he spoke of the friendship among Egyptian and American scientists who had "taken upon themselves to achieve one goal: the relief of the sufferings of mankind."[31] U.S. Ambassador Stanton Griffis in his speech stated dramatically that, only three years after the end of World War II, armies were again on the march. But, he said, another army, an international army, dressed in white and armed with microscopes and X-rays, with vaccines, and with constantly increasing medical knowledge was fighting for the health, dignity, and goodwill of the world. This army was winning on every front. While he acknowledged that the governments of Egypt and the United States differed in political viewpoints, he believed that "the great heart of Egypt" would never forget the efforts that the United States had made to help during the recent cholera epidemic, nor would the goodwill of Egypt toward the United States be seriously hurt if institutions like NAMRU-3 continued. In turn, he stated, the affection of the United States for Egypt would never be changed by political arguments.

Al-Siyasa, published by the Liberal Constitutionalist party, commented bitterly on the American ambassador's speech. It said that Egypt had indeed not forgotten that the United States had helped during the cholera epidemic with advice and vaccines, but that help did not mean that Egypt should compromise itself for aid that had taken place at a time different from the present. Egypt, it continued, had appealed to the world to help the Palestinian refugees, but the only American response had come from private humanitarian organizations connected with the international agencies. Egyptians welcomed cooperation between Egypt and the United States, but they did not want such cooperation to be like that between man and sheep: "Man gives food and water to the sheep to fatten it up before he slaughters it."[32] Despite the negative public reaction, NAMRU-3 continued to operate in Egypt. It carried out its research programs under the auspices of the Ministry of Health, and numerous Egyptian students and research scientists utilized its library and laboratory facilities. In the coming years, American involvement in Egypt's public health establishment was to broaden.

Meanwhile the palace announced that open elections for a new government would be held in late 1949. The Wafd, which had been out of power since October 1944, won the election and returned to power early in 1950 with new promises to deal with Egypt's social and economic problems. People hoped the Wafd, still the majority party, would finally carry out the long-promised reforms.[33] The new government lifted martial law and eased some of the political restrictions of the Sidqi, Nuqrashi, and Abd al-Hadi regimes. It passed legislation distributing a million feddans of state land to landless fellahin.[34] It passed several laws designed to improve social welfare and resumed Wakil's rural health unit program, but the reforms fell short of what had been promised.[35]

At the end of the 1940s talk of social upheaval and revolution was in the air. All efforts to dislodge the British troops had failed. Britain had prevented Egypt from maintaining hegemony over Sudan. Inflation continued, the wealthy Egyptian and foreign elites continued to enrich themselves, and labor strikes grew increasingly militant. In 1948–49 Egypt had been engulfed and defeated in the Palestine War. King Faruq and the palace were thoroughly discredited for their flagrant corruption. Anti-British demonstrations continued. The atmosphere of fear and instability intensified when Egyptian guerrillas began to attack British troops, which were still stationed in the Suez Canal region.[36]

On 25 January 1952 British troops surrounded an auxiliary Egyptian police station in Ismailia. The British believed that some of the Egyptian police officers inside had protected guerrillas who were responsible for terrorist attacks against British installations. The minister of the interior gave orders to the police not to surrender. British tanks and artillery then bombarded the barracks, while the men inside followed their orders. When they finally did surrender, after resisting for many hours, fifty-two men had died. The next day crowds ran through Cairo burning British hotels and clubs. The rioting spread, and thousands of foreign-owned businesses were burned. The palace, hoping to implicate the Wafd government, did nothing; the Wafd government, hoping to implicate the palace, did nothing. Finally after hours of rioting and extensive destruction, Faruq ordered the army to restore order. The inertia of the Wafd government and the palace and the British attack on the police station completed the discrediting of all three.

On the night of 22–23 July 1952 a group of disaffected army officers, who called themselves the Free Officers, seized power in a nearly bloodless military coup d'état. The Free Officers had diverse, nonelite but not impoverished backgrounds. Like most military men, they believed in ruling with a firm hand and in reforming Egypt from the top down. As a group they had no clear ideology other than their nationalism and their wish to reform Egypt, though some were attracted to Marxist ideas or to the Muslim Brotherhood's ideas or to both. In his famous pamphlet, *The Philosophy of the Revolution,* Gamal Abd al-Nasser, who soon emerged as the leader of the Free Officers, stated, "Every people on earth goes through two revolutions: a political revolution by which it wrests the right to govern itself from the hand of tyranny or from the army stationed upon its soil against its will; and a social revolution, involving the conflict of classes, which settles down when justice is secured for the citizens of the united nation." The pamphlet, published after the coup, implied that the Free Officers would now lead Egypt through both revolutions at once.[37]

Soon after the coup, Nur al-Din Tarraf, the physician and Hizb al-Watani party leader who had made the outspoken criticisms during the Chamber of Deputies interpellation about the government's handling of the cholera epidemic, became minister of health. In a newspaper interview, Tarraf stated that the improvement of the standard of health was to be a government priority because healthy individuals are better producers and so contribute more to the national income. A new generation of doctors would live in the villages, mix with the inhabitants, and become "pillars of health and social reform."[38] Indeed, there was much to be done. As seen above, in 1952 only 205 of the 860 rural health units and only 136 rural social centers had been built.[39] Many were little more than empty buildings. Unlicensed indigenous practitioners provided most of the health care but were not included or, with the exception of the *daya*s, even mentioned in governmental public health policy statements.

In 1953 the Free Officers established the Permanent Council for Public Welfare Services. The council drew up a five-year plan (1955–60) according to which the rural health units established in the 1940s would become part of new and larger "combined units." Each unit was to contain a health center, a school, and an agricultural and social services facility housed in three separate buildings on a five-feddan lot. The plan for combined units stated that public-welfare services should not be considered the responsibility of private charity because they were essential for social stability and for economic progress.[40] In 1955 Gamal Abd al-Nasser, who had emerged as head of state, himself opened the first combined unit.[41] The original plan was to build 600 units in five years, with the number of units later expanded to 868. The program was not innovative, rather it was a modification of the rural health unit and social center programs begun by Abd al-Wahid al-Wakil in 1942 and by Ismail Sidqi in 1946. The earlier type of rural health units and social centers also continued to function, and new units were built in the 1950s and 1960s.[42] In 1956 the rural health units and combined centers reported about three and one-half million outpatient visits and about eleven thousand hospital admissions.[43]

By the mid-1950s the Mabarra Muhammad Ali and the Women's Committee of the Red Crescent Association had become well-established medical assistance societies running hospitals, clinics, and emergency relief programs.[44] Hidiya Afifi Barakat was president of the Mabarra, which had 103 full-time male workers, 76 full-time female workers, and about 22 volunteers. According to its listing in the *Directory of Social Agencies in Cairo,* it had served "409,975 people of all nationalities, all religions, all ages and of both sexes, consisting of needy people and people of diverse occupations."[45] Mrs. Abd al-Hamid Shawarbi was president of the Women's Committee of the Red Crescent Association, which had three full-time male workers and about eighteen volunteers. In the listing it reported that it was serving in 1956 "4,955 people of all nationalities and religions, of all ages and of both sexes, consisting of underprivileged families as well as people of diverse occupations."[46] In addition, the directory lists over a hundred charitable organizations that provided medical services to the needy. The following listings suggest the diversity of the organizations: the First-Aid Public Assistance Association; the Great Coptic Benevolent Association; the Jewish Community Benevolent Association; the Kitchener Memorial Society (Hospital); the Lady Cromer Dispensaries for Sick Children; the Maraa el Gedida Association (the New Woman); the al-Shar'ia Association for the Followers of the Koran and the Mohammedan Sunna; the Tahrir Social Welfare Association; and the Egyptian Women's Union. The Mabarra Muhammad Ali and the Women's Committee of the Red Crescent Association were by far the most active and visible of the groups that provided large-scale emergency public relief and medical services. In 1950, Ahmad Hussayn, the minister of social affairs, estimated that some quarter million volunteers served in about three thousand charitable societies.[47]

In 1956 the government promulgated Law No. 384 of 1956, which brought all private societies and foundations dealing with social welfare under close governmental supervision.[48] In the early 1960s the Mabarra Muhammad Ali's hospitals and clinics were nationalized. Hidiya Afifi Barakat, the Mabarra's most active organizer, was the only volunteer to stay on to work under the government's administration of the Mabarra's hospitals and clinics. In 1969, on the last day of her life, she received Egypt's First Class Order of Merit for public service. Three years later, in November 1972, Mary Kahil was also decorated for her many years of philanthropy. Abla Sa'id Ahmad, the Mabarra nurse who served in Upper Egypt in 1944, stayed on and was nursing supervisor in the 1980s. The Red Crescent hospital and other facilities were also nationalized, but because the organization was connected to the International Red Cross, it was able to function with little governmental control—though without the patronage of members of the royal family.

The Mabarra Muhammad Ali and the Red Crescent were, of course, especially suspect to the new government because of their close association with the palace and the wealthy elite. But charitable organizations in general did not fare well under the new government; the government considered the benefits given by charity to be a basic right and an obligation of the government, and it sought to establish its control at all levels of society. In effect, Law No. 384 of 1956 limited private initiative in philanthropic activity and deprived Egypt of a valuable resource in public health care. While many women found increased opportunities in government-sponsored higher education and in certain professions, the volunteer women were suddenly removed from what had become, for many, their central occupation. By all accounts the standards in the Mabarra hospitals and clinics suffered when they came under governmental administration. The government personnel tended to lack experience and the devotion to public service that had motivated most of the volunteers.[49]

In July 1959 a presidential decree decentralized the Ministry of Health. Each of Egypt's twenty governorates was to have its own public-health administration.[50] Public health reformers had long complained that the rural health services suffered from being administrated by several ministries and departments at once and that administration from Cairo had resulted in bureaucratic confusion, delays, and faulty decisions. But decentralization was never fully implemented, and the officials in Cairo continued to dictate public-health administration.

While the government curtailed the activities of domestic organizations, such as the Mabarra Muhammad Ali and the Red Crescent, it was willing to accept assistance from the American and other foreign governments and from private voluntary organizations. A year before the Free Officers' coup, the United States had agreed to give Egypt economic and technical assistance under the Point Four program.

In point four of his inaugural address of 20 January 1949, President Truman announced that the United States would "embark on a bold new program for making the benefits of our scientific advances and industrial progress available for the improvement and growth of underdeveloped areas."[51] The Point Four program was intended to encourage formerly colonized nations to avoid the example of China and to choose capitalist economic models rather than socialist or communist ones.

In 1951, Egypt and the United States, in their General Agreement for Technical Cooperation, agreed to exchange technical knowledge and skills to further develop Egypt's economy. Health was one area in which assistance was to be given. The new Free Officers' government welcomed the Point Four program, and in 1953 the Egyptian-American Rural Improvement Service (EARIS) was established. The goals of EARIS were to reclaim eighty thousand feddans of land in Buhayra and Fayum provinces, to build model villages, and to develop agricultural, educational, and medical services. Plans to build the Aswan High Dam, which would greatly expand Egypt's irrigation system, were underway, and the project leaders hoped to create a model for building new villages on the reclaimed land. An Egyptian-American joint committee was formed to develop clinical, preventive health, and sanitation services for the model villages.[52] About five thousand families were resettled on land reclaimed by the EARIS project, mostly in the Abis region of Buhayra province. The new village houses had pure running water and toilet facilities. Clinics and hospitals were well equipped. Yet there was poor sanitation, noted by all visitors, which was ascribed by project administrators to a lack of motivation on the part of the villagers. Nevertheless animals were removed from homes to animal shelters outside the villages (whenever available) despite the long-standing custom.[53] The project was suspended with the Suez Crisis of 1956, was restarted in the early 1960s, and came to an end with the deterioration of Egyptian-American political relations in 1965. The families stayed on the reclaimed land, but the villages were soon indistinguishable from other villages in the region.

The Point Four project was beset with political tensions. In an unpublished analysis, Hrair Dekmajian, a political scientist specializing in the Middle East, comments that "the powerful force of Egyptian nationalism directed at the lingering British presence, the reformist idealism of the military elite around Nasser, the U.S. determination to 'woo Egypt' at practically any cost, [the] pervasive Egyptian 'phobia' of avoiding any outside domination or direction, and the tendency to reject the substitution of U.S. domination for British domination" had prevented the implementation of many of the EARIS plans.[54]

American influence in Egypt's public-health institutions nevertheless continued to increase. The government in 1955 established the High Institute for Public Health in Alexandria with courses in public-health administration, statistics, sanitary engineering, health education, and epidemiology. Experts from the School of Public Health of the University of California, Berkeley, helped design the curriculum with funds from the U.S. Foreign Operations Administration.[55]

NAMRU-3 continued to prosper in Egypt. While the U.S. Navy owned and ran the facility, it continued to function under the auspices of the Egyptian Ministry of Health. Ali Tawfiq Shusha was made honorary director and consultant. Aside from about ten administrators and medical researchers from the U.S. Navy, all of the personnel were Egyptian. Many of Egypt's medical researchers trained at NAMRU-3, and students frequently studied at its excellent library.[56]

It is not clear what the attitude of the Free Officers would have been to the Rockefeller Foundation's activities in Egypt because, only two weeks before the coup, the foundation had pulled out of Egypt. This withdrawal was the result of a policy change made at the foundation's headquarters in New York that led to its worldwide de-emphasis on public health. The foundation had long been interested in scientific and technical solutions to human misery. At the beginning of the twentieth century the discovery of the role of vectors in disease transmission and of pesticides had seemed an ideal way to stamp out such diseases as malaria and hookworm, diseases that had plagued humanity for millennia. By the early 1950s, however, foundation experts had concluded that improving public health required political and social change rather than scientific or technical intervention. Meanwhile new high-yield wheat and other crops that had been developed in recent years seemed to promise new technical solutions to the problem of food shortages in Africa, Asia, and Latin America. The foundation therefore shifted its international programs from public health to agriculture and disbanded its International Health Division in Egypt and elsewhere.

After 1952 the World Health Organization continued to carry out medical and public health projects from its Eastern Mediterranean Regional Office, headquartered in Alexandria. British bilateral and private voluntary organizations also gave assistance, as did those of many other nations.

In 1962 the Egyptian government sponsored a film about the 1947 cholera epidemic. The film was made by Tawfiq Salah, a well-known progressive film director, and was entitled *Sira' al-abtal* (*Struggle of Heroes*). It starred Shukri Sarhan, Samira Ahmad, and Layla Tahir, all famous actors of the era. In the film, a young doctor begins his practice in a rural town located next to a British base. The local landlord lives a life of indulgence, while the poor sort through garbage thrown from the base. The new doctor attempts to introduce modern medical practices but meets resistance from the local midwife and the health inspector, who are threatened by his new ideas. While the conflict builds, a British soldier suddenly falls sick. Soon a mysterious disease is spreading through the town. The health inspector and the midwife try to block the doctor's efforts to identify the disease. Just in the nick of time the doctor overcomes his opposition, convinces the unresponsive authorities in Cairo that the disease is cholera, and assistance arrives. The young doctor is successful in his confrontation with the villains: the wealthy landlords, the British troops, the poorly trained medical practitioners, and the inefficient government bureaucracy. The film, which proved to be very popular and was seen by hundreds of thousands of people, used the cholera epidemic to illustrate Egypt's struggles against its clearly identified enemies. Public health had become an idiom in the national discourse.

The year the film was made the government promulgated its charter that stated, "The first right of all citizens is health care—not the bare treatment and drugs like goods bought and sold, but rather the unconditional guarantee of this care to every citizen in every corner of the country under conditions of comfort and service."[57] Public health had become a basic obligation of the government and a guaranteed right of its citizens.

Did the Free Officers succeed in carrying out the long-promised public health reforms? James Mayfield and Raymond Baker, American political scientists who specialize in contemporary Egypt, have argued that the "trumpeted" reforms began with "great fanfare and optimism" but fell far short of their stated goals.[58] In 1965 259 of the rural health units and 300 of the combined units were in operation. Because of the shortage, the government introduced the smaller "rural unit," which had no inpatient facilities and a limited staff.[59] Mayfield cites a 1965 survey conducted by Egypt's Institute of National Planning, which found that about 76 percent of males and 61 percent of females in villages with health centers (i.e., 1,525 out of 5,000 villages) had utilized the health services at least once.[60] The consensus was that the services, even when available, were inadequate. Baker cites a Soviet study that, based on official Egyptian figures, found that 18 percent of Egypt's rural population had received medical treatment in the government's rural health centers and notes that these government figures were likely to have been inflated as evidence of hard work.[61] He further cites a 1966 survey of Egypt's administrative structure published by *al-Ishtiraki,* a government-sponsored newspaper. The survey found that, in the rural health unit, "the physician who provides medical treatment is also frequently the responsible administrative official. He has to examine the patients and supervise the care given to mothers and children, health care in schools, and health inspection. He [has] to take care of recording deaths and births and to distribute drugs. He is responsible for taking care of the drug supplies and [for] delivering prescriptions to the patients."[62] This survey reached the same conclusions regarding excessive work load as had John Weir's survey made twenty years before. The pattern of centralized bureaucratic control had not been broken. Mayfield has argued that the inadequacy of the health services was due largely "to the attitudes and assumptions that both the peasant and the village official" had "toward each other" because the traditional families continued to dominate, and many village officials loathed their time away from Cairo.[63] Baker has suggested that the medical personnel were not sufficiently motivated to serve efficiently in the government's rural health centers.[64]

More significantly, however, despite claims of revolutionary change, the post-1952 government retained not only the public health structures and policies of the previous governments but also the underlying assumptions and ideas that had formed those structures and policies. Although medical and public health facilities were substantially expanded, the governmental solutions to public health problems remained authoritarian and technocratic. With the benefit of forty years' hindsight and experience with development strategies worked out by the World Health Organization and other agencies, one may conclude that Egypt's political leaders, before and after the 1952 coup, would have done well to work not only toward the redistribution of resources and of medical, educational, and social services but also toward increased popular participation in the formation of public health policy.

Nevertheless the reforms in medical services, sanitation, land reform, income distribution, and education that were begun in the 1940s and expanded in the 1950s and later years all contributed to vastly improved health indexes.[65] As seen above, average life expectancy in 1942 had been thirty-one years for men and thirty-six years for women. In 1975 the average life expectancy at birth was about fifty-two years for men and fifty-five years for women.[66] Much remained to be done, but the foundation for further public health struggles had been laid.

10

Conclusion

The participants in Egypt's public-health wars had launched a major mobilization of human and material resources. Many lessons were learned during the campaigns against malaria, relapsing fever, and cholera. The combination of public and private initiative, of government and volunteer workers, of domestic and international expertise, and of open political competition and popular struggle proved effective against the biological invaders. The field of epidemiology, developed in Egypt by A. M. Kamal, the director of preventive medicine during the cholera epidemic, became an integral part of the curriculum of the new High Institute for Public Health. New methods for controlling epidemic diseases were adopted by the Ministry of Health and, while disease continues to afflict the populace, no large-scale epidemics have occurred since the 1940s. Falciparum malaria has reappeared sporadically in Egypt, as it has in Brazil, but each time the *Anopheles gambiae* mosquito has been diligently eradicated.

During the malaria epidemic Sadallah Madwar, Muhyi al-Din Farid, and the other Ministry of Health experts made a valiant effort to cope with the emergency despite their lack of resources. The volunteer women's missions assisted thousands of malaria victims and brought the disaster to the nation's attention. King Faruq made public health an area of personal interest following his birthday visit to Upper Egypt. In subsequent years he continued to associate himself with public health reform programs. The rivalries among the palace, the Wafd, and the British and the parliamentary debates not only stimulated efforts to deal with the epidemics but further emphasized the new political importance of public health reform. Under pressure from the palace and the British embassy, the Wafd government invited the Rockefeller Foundation to carry out an eradication campaign. Its success was countered by a British attempt to regain preeminence in public health.

The British-American rivalry was complicated by the appearance of yet another American organization, the U.S. Navy's NAMRU-3. The establishment of this medical research unit in Egypt eliminated British hopes of establishing one themselves. The technocratic approach of the American agencies reinforced an existing tendency to view public health reform as a technical and engineering challenge rather than as a political, social, and economic problem and to rely on bureaucratic administrative decisions rather than on popular participation in reforming public health policies. The technical expertise that the foreign experts brought to Egypt, however, proved invaluable in dealing with later epidemic diseases and with endemic public health problems.

During the relapsing fever epidemic the British and the Americans competed in supplying DDT and other materials that enabled the Ministry of Health, assisted by the volunteer women and the international health workers, to bring the epidemic to an end. Once again political rivalry had accelerated the epidemic control work, and the combination of efforts by many groups within Egyptian society resulted in an effective public-health campaign.

When cholera struck, the Mahmud Fahmi al-Nuqrashi government—remembering the attempts by the Mustafa Nahhas government to conceal the malaria epidemic—immediately allowed extensive media coverage. Volunteers from the Mabarra Muhammad Ali, the Red Crescent, the Wafd, the Muslim Brotherhood, Haditu, Young Egypt, and the wealthy elite all attempted to help. The international effort to supply Egypt with anticholera vaccine was a massive undertaking that enabled the Ministry of Health to vaccinate its entire population. It was the first time in history that such a campaign had been carried out. The national mobilization, the evident link between cholera and poverty, and the possibility of a British connection in the introduction of the disease into Egypt firmly and irrevocably placed public health in the political arena. The epidemic flamed nationalistic sentiment and reactivated calls for internal reform.

In response to the epidemics the contenders for power in Egypt intensified their efforts to carry out the long-promised reforms. While considerable progress was made, public health conditions remained in urgent need of improvement. Following the 1952 coup the Free Officers vowed to carry out the reforms themselves. In their quest for better health they often confronted many of the same political, social, and economic obstacles that had been confronted by their predecessors, but they managed to expand the programs and to increase access to medical and public-health facilities. Their programs were derived from programs begun by the Ministry of Social Affairs in the late 1930s and especially by Abd al-Wahid al-Wakil and the Wafd government in the early 1940s. They were much aided not only by the recent experiences of Egypt's public health officials but also by the new popular awareness of the crucial importance of improved public health. The campaigns against malaria, relapsing fever, and cholera had made public health in its widest sense a central part of Egypt's nationalist struggle. In future years public health policymakers would continue to be influenced by the ideas and attitudes formed during the public health wars of the 1940s.

Notes

Bibliography

Index

Notes

1. Introduction

1. For general information on diseases in the Middle East in the 1940s see E. B. Worthington, *Middle East Science: A Survey of Subjects Other than Agriculture* (London: H. M. Stationery Office, 1946), 140–57.

2. Robert Berkow, *The Merck Manual of Diagnosis and Therapy*, 15th ed. (Rahway, N.J.: Merck Sharp & Dohme Research Laboratories, 1987), 205–8.

3. Worthington, 142.

4. The World Health Organization considers malaria the primary health threat to international travelers. Chloroquine remains the standard prophylactic in Central America, India, parts of China, and western and central Africa, but in East Africa, northern South America, and Southeast Asia, chloroquine-resistant malaria exists. In addition, mosquitoes resistant to DDT and other insecticides are spreading in many regions. Medical researchers are currently using genetic engineering to develop antimalarial vaccines.

5. Relapsing fever, which is also called *recurrent fever*, is also transmitted by ticks in Europe, Asia, and parts of North and South America.

6. Berkow, 132–34.

7. For a history of the development of cholera vaccines see R. Pollitzer, *Cholera* (Geneva: World Health Organization, 1959), 263ff; and W. E. van Heyningen and John R. Seal, *Cholera: The American Scientific Experience, 1947–1980* (Boulder, Colo.: Westview, 1983), 151–213.

8. Ibid., 151–56.

9. van Heyningen and Seal, 157–68.

10. For information on public health development in Egypt and on the epidemics of cholera and plague in the nineteenth century, see LaVerne Kuhnke, *Lives at Risk: Public Health in Nineteenth-Century Egypt* (Berkeley: Univ. of California Press, 1989); and Robert L. Tignor, "Public Health Administration in Egypt under British Rule, 1882–1914" (Ph.D. diss., Yale Univ., 1960).

11. United Kingdom, *House of Commons Parliamentary Papers,* State Papers, Egypt 89, 1884–85, Report by H. R. Greene, Feb. 1885, Cairo, 75–76.

12. Traditional methods were often modified by acquaintance with modern medicine. For information on traditional medicine, see Hamed Ammar, *Growing Up in an Egyptian Village: Silwa, Province of Aswan* (London: Routledge & Kegan, 1954), 78ff; and John Walker, *Folk Medicine in Modern Egypt* (London: Luzac, 1934). This book was written by Abd al-Rahman Ismail, a physician at

Qasr al-Ayni hospital, and published in Cairo in 1892–94. Ismail hoped to replace the earlier practices with modern ones. An interesting but much earlier source is Pierre-Charles Rouyer, "Notice sur les médicamens usuels des Egyptiens," in *Description de l'Egypte,* état moderne 10 (Paris: l'Imprimerie Impériale, 1809), 217–32. Rouyer's account is discussed in J. Worth Estes and LaVerne Kuhnke, "French Observations of Disease and Drug Use in Late Eighteenth-Century Cairo," *Journal of the History of Medicine and Allied Sciences,* 39, no. 2 (Apr. 1984): 121–52. For a survey of ethnographic literature, see Barbara Pillsbury, *Traditional Health Care in the Near East* (Washington, D.C.: U.S. Agency for International Development, 1983), 22–61. See also Serge Jagailloux, "Médecines et santé dans l'Egypte du XIXe siècle" (doc. d'état: Univ. of Paris IV, Sorbonne, 1983).

13. Winifred Blackman cited a cure for fever in which a *shaykh* known for his healing powers would inscribe with a reed pen "Hell is hot, cold, thirsty, and hungry" on four pieces of paper, then put seven seeds of cumin on each piece of paper, wrap the papers around pieces of candle, and tie them with spider's web. In an attack of fever, the patient would dip the roll of paper in olive oil, place the roll in a bowl, and burn it so that the fumes would permeate his or her clothing. With each attack the patient burned a roll until the fever was cured (Winifred Blackman, *The Fellahin of Upper Egypt* [London: Harrap, 1927], 206–7).

14. For a brief description of the evil eye in Nubia, see Robert Fernea, *Nubians in Egypt: Peaceful People* (Austin: Univ. of Texas Press, 1973), 24.

15. Personal communication, Salih Marafi, Luxor.

16. Personal communication, Salah Attiyya, Alexandria.

17. This attitude, despite a certain appreciation for the recent interest in medical anthropology and social medicine, has largely dominated public health policymaking to the present.

18. Tignor, "Public Health Administration," 136–38; Kuhnke, 120–21.

19. Kuhnke, 72.

20. A. Milner, *England in Egypt* (London: E. Arnold, 1920), 293.

21. Ibid., 293–94.

22. *British Medical Journal* 1 (March 1951): 688. The actual figure was probably about one hundred thousand (Robert L. Tignor, *Modernization and British Colonial Rule in Egypt, 1882–1914* [Princeton: Princeton Univ. Press, 1986], 349; Tignor, "Public Health Administration," 84–87).

23. Tignor, "Public Health Administration," 63.

24. *The British Medical Journal* gives 16,571 officially reported deaths from cholera in 1895–96 (*British Medical Journal* 1 [Mar. 1951]): 688. Pollitzer gives 16,000 cholera deaths for 1895–96 and 34,000 for 1902 (Pollitzer, 40–42). For an Egyptian physician's account of the 1902 cholera epidemic, see Naguib Mahfouz, The Life of an Egyptian Doctor (Edinburgh and London: E. & S. Livingston, Ltd., 1956), 38–54.

25. Neville Goodman, *International Health Organizations and Their Work* (London: J. & A. Churchill, 1951), 5–8, 51–54, 61–64.

26. Tignor, "Public Health Administration," 99–100; M. Khalil, "The Defence of Egypt against Cholera in the Past, Present, and Future," *Journal of the Royal Egyptian Medical Association* 30 (Dec. 1947): 620–21. For a history of the Egyptian quarantine service, see Kuhnke, 92–109.

27. Tignor, "Public Health Administration," 78.

28. Ibid., 60.

29. Lord Cromer, *Modern Egypt* (London: Macmillan and Co., 1908), 860–61.

30. United Kingdom, *House of Commons Parliamentary Papers*, Egypt, Cd. 3394, 100, 1907, 96–97. See also "Medicine in the Land of Pharoes, Ancient and Modern," *Journal of the Egyptian Medical Association* 11, no. 10 (Dec. 1928): 356 J; and Tignor, *Modernization*, 331–33.

31. "Medicine in the Land of Pharoes, Ancient and Modern," *Journal of the Egyptian Medical Association* 11, 10 (Dec. 1928), 356 J–356 K.

32. Mahfouz Naguib, *The History of Medical Education in Egypt* (Cairo: Government Press at Bulaq, 1935), 54–61.

33. For further information on the medical profession see Amira El Azhary Sonbol, "The Creation of a Medical Profession in Egypt during the Nineteenth Century: A Study in Modernization" (Ph.D. diss., Georgetown Univ., 1981).

34. Mahfouz Naguib, *History of Medical Education*, 71–76; Kuhnke, 122–33.

35. Tignor, *Modernization*, 354.

36. Ibid., 356.

37. *Mabarra al-Mar'at al-jadida.* (Cairo: n.p., n.d.) brochure. Huda Sha'rawi describes the origins and early years of the Mabarra Muhammad Ali in her memoirs (*Harem Years: The Memoirs of an Egyptian Feminist, 1879–1924*. Margot Badran trans. and intro. [London: Virago Press, 1986], 94–98).

38. Isis Istiphan, *Directory of Social Agencies in Cairo* (Cairo: American Univ. at Cairo, 1956), 211.

39. E. Richard Brown, *Rockefeller Medicine Men: Medicine and Capitalism in America* (Berkeley: Univ. of California Press, 1979), 112.

40. Ibid., 113.

41. Ibid., 119, 123.

42. Gordon Harrison, *Mosquitoes, Malaria, and Man: A History of the Hostilities since 1880* (New York: Dutton, 1978), 23–108. For a brief discussion of malaria in pre–World War I Egypt, see Tignor, "Public Health Administration," 97–100.

43. Raymond B. Fosdick, *The Story of the Rockefeller Foundation* (London: Odhams, 1952), 14–43.

44. Brown, 129ff.

45. Fosdick, 37. For a discussion of how the antimalarial program in Latin America served the economic interests of the Rockefeller Foundation, see Saul Franco-Agudelo, "The Rockefeller Foundation's Antimalaria Program in Latin America: Donating or Dominating?" *International Journal of Health Services* 13, no. 1 (1983): 51–67.

46. Egypt, Hookworm Disease, Approval of Project, 18 Jan. 1928, RG 1.1, Series 485 H, RFA.

47. Memo on Ankylostoma and Bilharzia Control, submitted by Catheart Garner, Colonel Director General to Director General, 9 May 1920, RG 5, Series 2, Special Reports, RFA.

48. Marius Deeb, *Party Politics in Egypt: The Wafd and Its Rivals, 1936–1939* (London: Ithaca Press, 1979), 272.

49. For the early history of the Department of Public Health, see D. M. Siba'i (D. M. Sebai), "History of the Evolution of the Department of Public Health in Egypt," *Journal of the Egyptian Medical Association* 11, no. 10 (Dec. 1928): 357–67.

50. For a brief history of the Ministry of Social Affairs, see Ahmed Hussein, *Social Welfare in Egypt* (Cairo: Ministry of Social Welfare, 1950).

51. The cooperative movement in Egypt is traced to the formation of cooperative societies by Umar Lutfi in 1908 (Ahmed Hussein, *Social Welfare,* 41–59).

52. Ahmed Hussein, *Social Welfare,* 82–83.

53. Ahmed Zaher Zaghloul, "Rural Health Services in U.A.R.," *Journal of the Egyptian Public Health Association* 38, no. 5 (1963): 220–24.

54. A. J. Warren to Major Lundeberg, 23 July 1941, RG 2, Series 475, Box 223, RFA.

55. Ibid.

56. For further discussion of the 1936 Treaty, see Mahmud Y. Zayid, *Egypt's Struggle for Independence* (Beirut: Khayats, 1965), 135–90.

57. Martin W. Wilmington, *The Middle East Supply Centre* (Albany: State Univ. of New York Press, 1971), 14.

58. Ibid., 238 (map). The map shows the enormous size of British military training areas delimited by the 1936 Treaty.

59. Jacques Berque, *Egypt: Imperialism and Revolution,* Jean Stewart, trans. (London: Faber, 1972), 569.

60. Declaration by Prominent Egyptians in Advocacy of Social Reform Measures, 23 Jan. 1941, RG 59, File 883.12/93, NA.

61. Wilmington, 22–25; P. J. Vatikiotis, *The Modern History of Egypt* (Baltimore: Johns Hopkins Univ. Press, 1985), 347–48.

62. Kirk to Secretary of State, 15 Feb. 1944, RG 84, Box 110, 812.1, NA.

63. For further information on Faruq, see Barrie St. Clair McBride, *Farouk of Egypt* (London: Robert Hale, 1967).

64. W. Roger Louis, *The British Empire in the Middle East, 1945–1951: Arab Nationalism, the United States, and Postwar Imperialism* (New York: Oxford Univ. Press, 1984), 49.

65. The advance of Italian and German troops led Egyptian leaders, including Faruq, to hedge their bets and support a government friendly to both the Axis and the Allies. On 2 February 1942, Prime Minister Husayn Sirri, who was pro-British, had resigned. The deteriorating economic, political, and military conditions and the palace's opposition to his breaking relations with Pe-

tain's France had led to his resignation. Faruq had planned to ask Ali Mahir, who had been prime minister before Sirri, to form a government of mostly palace officials whom the British suspected of harboring pro-Axis sympathies.

66. Michael Wright to Hankey, 27 Feb. 1942, FO 141/850.

67. Ibid.

68. Health: Condition of in Egypt, 27 Feb.–12 Mar. 1942, FO 141/850.

69. See Thomas Russell, *Egyptian Service, 1902–1946* (London: Murray, 1949), 35–41.

70. Health: Conditions of in Egypt, 27 Feb.–12 Mar. 1942, FO 141/850.

2. Malaria Invades

1. The population of Nubia was about fifty-five thousand in 1944.

2. Ali Tawfiq Shusha (Aly Tewfik Shousha), "Species-Eradication: The Eradication of the *Anopheles gambiae* from Upper Egypt, 1942–1945," *Bulletin of the World Health Organization* 1, no. 2 (1948): 312; Egypt, *Taqrir al-jambia* (Report on Gambiae) (Cairo: Ministry of Health, 1950), 1–4.

3. D. J. Lewis, "A Northern Record of *Anopheles gambiae*," *Royal Entomological Society of London Proceedings,* Series B 11 (1942): 141–42. The malaria expert who discovered the mosquito larvae was Dr. R. T. Campbell.

4. Siba'i, 361.

5. George Kirk, *The Middle East in the War* (London and New York: Oxford Univ. Press, 1952), 257–58.

6. Soper diary, 21 Jan. 1943.

7. Kerr diary, 19 July 1944; 20 Feb. 1945.

8. Ibid., 20 Feb. 1945.

9. Soper diary, 23 Mar. 1945.

10. D. J. Lewis, "The Control of Anopheles gambiae in the Wadi Halfa Area," 1 July 1943, FO 370/799; Soper diary, 23 Mar. 1945.

11. Muhyi al-Din Farid (Mohyeedin Ahmad Farid), "A Preliminary Note on An Unusual Breeding Place of *Anopheles gambiae* in Egypt," *Journal of the Egyptian Medical Association* 26, no. 4 (Apr. 1943): 126–27.

12. Personal communication, Myhyi al-Din Farid.

13. D. J. Lewis, "The Control of Anopheles gambiae in the Wadi Halfa Area," 1 July 1943, FO 370/799.

14. Kerr diary, 19 July 1944; personal communication, Muhyi al-Din Farid.

15. Shusha, "Species-Eradication," 340–41; Killearn to Eden, 31 May 1943, FO 370/799; J. Austin Kerr, ed., *Building the Health Bridge: Selections from the Works of Fred L. Soper* (Bloomington, Ind.: Indiana Univ. Press, 1970), 299. See also the discussion in Worthington, 143.

16. Japan had occupied Java in 1941, cutting off the world's supply of quinine, the standard antimalarial drug. Necessity being the mother of invention, the discovery of synthetic antimalarial drugs, such as chloroquine and Atabrine, soon followed. The synthetics were immediately produced on a large scale and proved more effective than quinine itself (Emilio Pampana, *A Textbook of Ma-*

laria Eradication [London and New York: Oxford Univ. Press, 1969], 243–44); Egypt, *Taqrir al-jambiyya*, 4–6.

17. Abd al-Fattah al-Tawil was minister of health from 6 February to 26 May 1942 followed by Wakil, who served from 26 May 1942 to 8 October 1944. For the tour of Upper Egypt, see *al-Ahram*, 22 Oct. 1942.

18. For more information on the incidence of these diseases, see chap. 8, n. 41.

19. *Al-Ahram*, 1 Dec. 1942.

20. Ibid., 9 Dec. 1942.

21. Sir Robin Furness Papers, Box 2, Private Papers Collection, Middle East Centre, St. Antony's College, Oxford.

22. The 1972 Nicaraguan earthquake, for example, strengthened the Sandinista movement and contributed to the fall of the Somoza regime in 1979 (Alan Riding, "Nicaragua: A National Mutiny?" *New York Times Sunday Magazine* [30 July 1978], 39–42). In Ethiopia royal disinterest in the Sahel famine contributed to the overthrow of Emperor Haile Selassie in 1974 (Jack Shepherd, *The Politics of Starvation* [New York: Carnegie Endowment for International Peace, 1975]; Rene Lefort, *Ethiopia: An Heretical Revolution?* [London: Zed Press, 1983]). The summer floods of 1974 exacerbated the unrest that ultimately toppled Mujibur Rahman, president of Bangladesh, in 1975 (Charles Peter O'Donnell, *Bangladesh: Biography of a Muslim Nation* [Boulder, Colo., Westview, 1984], 164–78). For a recent example, see "Politicians Often Tripped by Natural Disasters," *Los Angeles Times* (20 Oct. 1989), an article published following a major earthquake.

23. Wilmington, 14.

24. Harrison, 213–17.

25. Soper diary, 13 Jan. 1943.

26. Paris green (copper aceto-arsenite), an insecticide, was found to be effective against anopheline larvae in 1920. It was cheaper than Malariol; nontoxic to people, plants, fish, and cattle; and could easily be transported and mixed with dust at the site before being applied (Harrison, 186–87). Pyrethrum was derived from the powdered flowers of the chrysanthemum plant. Soper to Shusha, 25 Jan. 1943, RG 1.1, Series 485, Box 2, RFA; Fred L. Soper's report to Egyptian ministry of health, 25 Jan. 1943, FO 370/799. Soper was planning at the time to recommend the services of D. B. Wilson, a Canadian, and Dr. Paulo Antunes, a Brazilian, both of whom had worked in the Rockefeller Foundation's malaria service in Brazil.

27. Stephenson to Soper, RG 1.1, Series 485, Box 2, 5 Feb. 1943, RFA.

28. Ibid., 7 Feb. 1943, RFA.

29. Ibid.

30. Soper to Sawyer, 31 Jan. 1943, RG 1.1, Series 485, Box 2, RFA.

31. Soper to Sawyer, 11 Feb. 1943, Rockefeller Fondation Archives.

32. Soper to Wilson, 2 June 1944, RG 1.1, Series 485, Box 2, Folder 16, RFA.

33. Sir M. Lampson (Lord Killearn) to Foreign Office, 16 Feb. 1943, FO 370/799.

34. Ministry of War Transport to Middle East Supply Centre, Cairo, 13 Apr. 1943, FO 370/799.

35. Middle East Supply Centre, Cairo to Ministry of War Transport, 20 May 1943, FO 370/799.

36. Wilmington notes that Allied and colonial officials often conflicted and that the colonial officials obstructed the war effort through their underrating the capacities of their subjects and their conservative economic policies (Wilmington, 28).

37. Kerr, *Building the Health Bridge*, 300.

38. Killearn to Eden, 21 May 1943, FO 371/35598.

39. Killearn to Eden, 31 May 1943, FO 370/799.

40. Ibid.

41. Ibid.

42. Memorandum by Sir W. Smart, FO 371/35598.

43. Smart counters, "our critics are inclined to forget the work which we have done through British doctors working with the Health Department of the Egyptian Government, through Sir Ernest Cassel's charitable enterprise, through the Giza Ophthalmic Laboratory, through Municipal improvements." Memorandum by Sir W. Smart, FO 371/35598.

44. Ibid.

45. Health Conditions in Egypt, 21 May 1943, FO 371/35598.

46. Killearn to Eden, 21 May 1943, FO 371/35598.

47. Maurice Peterson to Wilson Jameson, 23 July 1943, FO 371/35595.

48. *Al-Ahram,* 16 May 1943.

49. In addition, a medical survey undertaken in the early 1940s found that about 84 percent of the population of Kom Ombo was infected with bilharzia and about 24 percent with hookworm (Worthington, 153).

50. Fred L. Soper, "Notes Taken on Trip to Upper Egypt," 12 May 1944, Record Group 1.1, Series 485 I, Box 2, Folder 16, RFA.

51. Egypt, *Madhabit,* Chamber of Deputies, session of 29 Feb. 1944, 773–821.

52. Ibid., 14 May 1944.

53. Ibid., 15 May 1944.

54. Ibid.

55. Shusha, "Species-Eradication," 316.

56. Soper, "Trip to Upper Egypt," 14 May 1944, RFA.

57. *Al-Ahram,* 21 Sept. 1945.

58. A. A. Shawarby, A. H. Mahdi, and S. Kotla, "Protective Measures against *Anopheles Gambiae* Invasion to UAR," *Journal of the Egyptian Public Health Association* 42, no. 5 (1967): 194.

59. Henry Habib Ayrout, *The Egyptian Peasant* (Boston: Beacon Press, 1968), 75; Ammar, 81.

60. Personal communication, Abd al-Aziz Salah.

61. Madwar admitted to Soper that, when the government requested de-

tailed statistics on malaria cases and fatalities, he had been forced to make them up because none had been kept in the early stages of the epidemic.

62. M. Khalil, "The 1936 Treaty and the Effect of the Second World War on the Health of the Egyptian Nation," *The Journal of the Royal Egyptian Medical Association* 31, no. 1 (Jan. 1948): 2.

63. Shusha, "Species-Eradication," 309–52.

64. Kerr, *Building the Health Bridge,* 301; Egypt, *Madhabit,* Chamber of Deputies, session of 29 Feb. 1944, 775.

65. Soper diary, 16 May 1944.

66. Kirk to Secretary of State, 19 Feb. 1944, RG 84, Box 110, File 812.1, NA.

67. Kerr diary, 12 Feb. 1945.

68. *Ruz al-Yusuf,* 8 June 1944.

69. The number of doses of Atabrine was taken as the number of cases of malaria. The case fatality rate was assumed to be about 10 percent. Often, however, doses of Atabrine were distributed nearly at random, and case fatality rates varied greatly from region to region.

70. Kerr, *Building the Health Bridge,* 301.

71. Deaths from Malaria in Qina-Aswan, 22 Oct. 1944, FO 370/927.

72. Dr. Fuad Habid, director of Treatment Service at al-Sabi'a to Soper ("Trip to Upper Egypt," 14 May 1944), RFA.

73. *London Economist* article cited in *al-Ahram,* 21 Feb. 1943.

74. *Al-Ahram,* 20 Dec. 1943.

75. Harrison, 186–89; Soper diary, 21 Jan. 1943.

76. Soper diary, 22 Mar. 1945.

77. Soper, "Trip to Upper Egypt," 11 May 1944, RFA.

78. Soper to Wilson, 2 June 1944, RG 1.1, Series 485, Box 2, RFA.

79. Soper diary, 22 Mar. 1945; Soper, "Trip to Upper Egypt," 16 May 1944, RFA.

80. Ayrout gives a largely unsympathetic account of the doctor's plight in rural Egypt and a more understanding account of the fellahin's difficulties in seeking medical advice (Ayrout, 75–77).

81. Kerr diary, 13 Jan. 1945.

82. Ibid. No significant differences in medical beliefs or attitudes toward disease appeared among the Muslim and Coptic communities of Upper Egypt during the confrontation with malaria.

83. In one village near Giza far outside the malaria zone, the midwife and the health barber had a long-standing feud, a not unusual phenomenon given their built-in conflict of interest. When the midwife fell ill with typhoid and was taken to the Abbasiyya Fever Hospital, the barber reported that the midwife's husband, a gardener, was also ill. The gardener fled to his employer's garden where he hid himself. When a second man died the barber reported that malaria had broken out in the village. The Malaria Section sent a team to the village where it set up tents and disinfection equipment. The team then seized eighteen villagers, whom it insisted were infected with malaria, and

detained them. No diagnostic slides were made. Those who could pay a bribe were released. The rest were detained for about five days, whereupon they were also released. Then the gardener returned home thinking it was safe but was again reported by the barber. The *sahha* sent three policemen to arrest him. He took off his clothes and offered "to take on the lot, to show what a dying man could do when put to it." Finally he was taken away but returned fifteen minutes later saying "my illness got out of my purse and left me" (Kerr diary, 23 Nov. 1944).

84. Ammar, 79.

85. Kerr diary, 4 Nov. 1944.

86. *Egyptian Gazette,* 13 Oct. 1943; *al-Ahram,* 13 Oct. 1943.

87. *Al-Ahram,* 16 Nov. 1943.

88. Ibid.

89. Ibid., 20 Dec. 1943.

90. Ibid.

91. Ibid., 21 Dec. 1943.

3. Elite Women and King Faruq to the Rescue

1. *Al-Ahram,* 12 Jan. 1944.

2. Ibid., and 1 Feb. 1944.

3. Ibid., 22 Jan. 1944.

4. *Ithnayn wa Dunya,* 21 Jan. 1944.

5. Among the later Red Crescent volunteers were Sophie Butrus Ghali, whose son Butrus became minister of state for foreign affairs in 1977; Salha Aflatun, daughter of Muhammad Aflatun and granddaughter of Aflatun Pasha; Amina al-'Alayili, daughter of Ahmad Niyazi, judge of the mixed courts and wife of Yahya al-'Alayili, secretary general of the Kom Ombo Sugar Company; and Celine Cattaui, wife of Rene Cattaui, who was the director of the Kom Ombo Sugar Company, a member of Parliament, and a leader of the Egyptian Jewish community (*Ithnayn wa Dunya,* 27 Mar. 1944).

6. Personal Communication, Abla Sa'id Ahmad; *Mabarrat al-mar'at al-jadida* brochure.

7. Personal communication, Muhyi al-Din Farid.

8. *Ithnayn wa Dunya,* 31 Jan. 1944.

9. Ghali diary, 25 Jan. 1944.

10. Ibid., 25 and 29 Jan. 1944.

11. *Ruz al-Yusuf,* 8 June 1944.

12. Asma Halim, *Sitta Ayam fi Sa'id* (Cairo: The New Dawn Publishing House, 1944 [summarized by Ahmad Qasim Guda in *Ruz al-Yusuf,* 8 June 1944]). The booklet was also serialized in *al-Ahd al-Jadid* (Selma Botman, "Oppositional Politics in Egypt: The Communist Movement, 1936–1954" [Ph.D. diss., Harvard, 1984], 561–62).

13. *Progres egyptien,* 21 Jan. 1944.

14. *Al-Ahram,* 4 Feb. 1944; *Egyptian Gazette,* 4 Feb. 1944.

15. Bain to Bellm, 24 Jan. 1944, RG 84, Box 110, File 812.1, NA.

16. Killearn to Foreign Office, 12 Feb. 1944, FO 371/41326.

17. Hasan Yusuf, *al-Qasr wa duruhu fi al-siyasat al-misriyya, 1922–1952* (Cairo: Markaz al-dirasat al-siyasiya wa al-istratijiya, 1982), 167–68.

18. Ibid.

19. *Egyptian Gazette,* 11 Feb. 1944.

20. Ibid.

21. *Al-Musawwar,* 18 Feb. 1944.

22. *Ruz al-Yusuf,* 25 Feb. 1944.

23. *Al-Musawwar,* 25 Feb. 1944; *al-Ahram,* 11–18 Feb. 1944; *Ruz al-Yusuf,* 23 Mar. 1944.

24. *Ruz al-Yusuf,* 2 Mar. 1944.

25. Ibid.

26. The most important of these were the publications of Young Egypt, the Muslim Brotherhood, and the communist organizations.

27. *Progres egyptien,* 29 and 31 Jan., 2 Feb. 1944.

28. *Al-Misri,* 12 Feb. 1944.

29. Personal communication, Muhyi al-Din Farid. The criticisms in the Muslim Brotherhood publications became more vitriolic during the 1946 relapsing fever epidemic.

30. *La bourse egyptienne,* 31 Jan. 1944.

31. *Khutbah,* 18 Feb. 1947, Mirit Butrus Ghali trans. Private papers of Mirit Butrus Ghali, Cairo. It might be noted here that none of the volunteer women contracted malaria, partly because the epidemic had lost its severity when they began their work and partly because they were able to screen themselves and their living quarters effectively against the anopheles mosquito.

32. *Khutbah,* 18 Feb. 1947.

33. Killearn to Foreign Office, 23 Feb. 1944, FO 371/41326.

34. *Akhir Sa'a,* 27 Feb. 1944.

35. Ibid.

36. *Egyptian Gazette,* 17 Feb. 1944.

37. *Ruz al-Yusuf,* 2 Mar. 1944.

38. Kuhnke, 122–33.

39. Afaf Lutfi al-Sayyid Marsot, "Egypt's Revolutionary Gentlewomen," in *Women in the Muslim World,* ed. Lois Beck and Nikki Keddie (Cambridge, Mass.: Harvard Univ. Press, 1976), 261–76.

40. Nawal El Saadawi, *The Hidden Face of Eve: Women in the Arab World* (London: Zed Press, 1980), 176.

41. According to Margot Badran, who has edited and translated Sha'rawi's memoirs, she saw the Mabarra Muhammad Ali women off at the train station and sent Hawa Idris, her cousin and protégée, to represent her on the missions (Margot Badran, "Huda Sha'rawi and the Liberation of the Egyptian Woman" [Ph.D. diss., Oxford Univ., 1977], 294–97. I have not found Idris mentioned among the participants.

42. Wendy Kaminer, *Women Volunteering: The Pleasure, Pain, and Politics*

of Unpaid Work from 1830 to the Present (Garden City, N.Y.: Anchor Press, 1984); Susan A. Ostrander, *Women of the Upper Class* (Philadelphia: Temple Univ. Press, 1984).

43. Personal communication, Wadud Fayzi Musa.

44. Personal communication, Mustafa Amin.

4. Malaria in Politics

1. Killearn to Foreign Office, 12 Feb. 1944, FO 371/41326.

2. Killearn diary, 30 Dec. 1943.

3. Memorandum: Malaria Epidemic in Upper Egypt, 10 Jan. 1944, FO 370/927.

4. Killearn diary, 14 Jan. 1944.

5. Killearn to Foreign Office, 15 Feb. 1944, FO 371/41326.

6. Ibid.

7. Ibid.

8. Killearn diary, 14 Feb. 1944.

9. Ibid., 15 Feb. 1944.

10. Ibid.

11. Kirk to Secretary of State, 7 Mar. 1944, RG 84, Box 110, File 812.1, NA.

12. *Musawwar,* 25 Feb. 1944.

13. Killearn diary, 21 Jan. 1944.

14. Killearn to Foreign Office, 16 Feb. 1944, FO 371/41326; Yusuf, 168–69.

15. Ibid., 168.

16. Killearn to Foreign Office, 24 Feb. 1944, FO 371/41326.

17. *Egyptian Gazette,* 17 Feb. 1944.

18. Publicity Section, 19 Feb. 1944, FO 371/41327.

19. Killearn diary, 21 Feb. 1944.

20. Killearn to Foreign Office, 24 Feb. 1944, FO 371/41326.

21. Killearn diary, 21 Feb. 1944.

22. Killearn to Foreign Office, 27 Feb. 1944, FO 371/41327.

23. *Egyptian Gazette,* 27 Feb. 1944; Second Communiqué, FO 371/41327.

24. Killearn diary, 23 Feb. 1944.

25. Killearn to Foreign Office, 28 Feb. 1944, FO 371/41327.

26. Ibid.

27. *Egyptian Gazette,* 29 Feb. 1944.

28. Egypt, *Madhabit,* Chamber of Deputies, session of 28 Feb. 1944, 556ff.

29. Ibid., 758–59.

30. Ibid., 761.

31. Ibid., 766ff.

32. Ibid., 772.

33. Ibid.

34. In 1938 two Wafdist leaders, Mahmud Fahmi al-Nuqrashi and Ahmad Mahir, broke off to form the Saʿdist party, named after the founder of the Wafd party, Saʿd Zaghlul. Mahir and Nuqrashi had been active members of the Wafd

party since its inception following World War I, but they had come to disagree with the Wafd's inflexible anti-British policy. The Saʻdist party platform stated that its purpose was to restore the principles of the original Wafd party. Its members, who were mainly industrialists, businessmen, technicians, and managers, lacked the rural base of the Wafd party and were willing to work with the palace (Marius Deeb, *Party Politics in Egypt: The Wafd and Its Rivals, 1936–1939* [London: Ithaca Press, 1979], 246–48).

35. Egypt, *Madhabit*, Chamber of Deputies, session of 29 Feb. 1944, 773–821.

36. Ibid.

37. *Egyptian Gazette*, 1 Mar. 1944.

38. Egypt, *Madhabit*, Chamber of Deputies, session of 29 Feb. 1944, 773–821.

39. Marcel Colombe, *L'Évolution de l'Égypt, 1924–1950* (Paris: G. P. Maisonneuve, 1951), 112–13.

40. Killearn diary, 29 Feb. 1944.

41. Kirk to Secretary of State, 11 Mar. 1944, RG 84, Box 110, File 812.1, NA.

42. Killearn to Foreign Office, 2 Mar. 1944, FO 371/41327.

43. Ibid., 12 and 16 Mar. 1944.

44. Report on Malaria Control, submitted to Wakil, 6 Mar. 1944, and to Eden, 28 Mar. 1944, FO 370/927; Recommendations on Malaria Control in Upper Egypt, by Crawford and Caplan, 16 Mar. 1944, RG 84, Box 110, File 812.1, NA.

45. *Al-Misri*, 27 Mar. 1944.

46. *Ithnayn wa Dunya*, 7 Mar. 1944.

47. Ibid.

48. Ibid.

49. Ibid.

50. *Ruz al-Yusuf*, 30 Mar. 1944.

51. Ibid.

52. See, for example, *Ithnayn wa Dunya*, 8 Feb. 1944.

53. Quoted in Gabriel Baer, *A History of Land Ownership in Modern Egypt, 1800–1950* (London: Oxford Univ. Press, 1962), 203–4.

54. Egypt, *Annual Report on the Work of the Ministry of Public Health* (Cairo: Ministry of Public Health, 1944), 86.

55. Killearn to Eden, 15 Mar. 1944, FO 370/927.

56. The Kutla party was led by Makram Ebeid, who had been an active leader of the Wafd party until he became disillusioned by its corruption. In 1943 he had clandestinely prepared and circulated a "Black Book" documenting the excesses of the party. He then founded a separate opposition political party, Kutlat al-Wafd (Bloc of the Wafd party) or Kutla party.

57. *Al-Musawwar*, 7 Apr. 1944.

58. In 1922 a small group of disaffected Wafdists had broken away from the party and formed the Liberal Constitutionalist party. This party, which re-

mained small, was similar to the Wafd party in political ideology and membership. It was a party of wealthy landowners, while many Wafdists were middle-level landowners (Deeb, 75–80). The National party (*Hizb al-Watani*) was founded before World War I. It was eclipsed and suppressed by the Wafd party in the nationalistic struggles of the early 1920s. Muhammad Hafiz Ramadan became president of the party in 1923. It opposed the Wafd and called for ties with other Muslim nations of the Middle East (Deeb, 80–85).

59. The National Front, Second Call, 23 Mar. 1944, FO 371/41327.

60. Ibid.

61. Kirk to Secretary of State, 7 Apr. 1944, RG 84, Box 110, File 812.2, NA.

62. *Egyptian Gazette,* 31 Mar. 1944.

63. Ibid.; Kirk to Secretary of State, 11 Apr. 1944, RG 84, Box 110, File 812.2, NA.

64. *Al-Misri,* 2–6 Apr. 1944.

65. Kirk to Secretary of State, 7 Apr. 1944, RG 84, Box 110, File 812.2, NA.

66. In the fall of 1944, when the Wafd government was no longer in power, Makram Ebeid, the new minister of finance and founder of the Kutla party, was to charge the Wafd party with expropriating the funds collected for malaria relief and to demand the return of £E 140,500. He said that in April 1944, the Wafd's undersecretary for social affairs had withdrawn the money from Bank Misr, where the funds had been deposited. Nahhas explained that the money had been withdrawn for safekeeping because it appeared at the time that the government was about to fall. Makram Ebeid then asked why the government did not redeposit the money when conditions stabilized. Nahhas replied that the monies were not state funds but charitable donations, such as funds collected by the Red Crescent or the Islamic League and were deposited in the National Bank of Egypt in his name to be used to endow two orphanages in Upper Egypt. Ebeid answered that the money had been demanded by government officials, which was not the way private charities collected their funds. Furthermore, he said, the money had been collected to help the victims of malaria, not to build orphanages. After more dickering, Nahhas put the funds back in a new account in the name of the government, which then withdrew it (*al-Dustur,* 15 Oct. 1944; *al-Balagh,* 19 Oct. 1944; *Egyptian Gazette,* 19 Dec. 1944; *al-Ahram,* 22 Dec. 1944). In this way the new regime attempted to discredit the former Wafdist officials, who, for their part, considered their money to have been expropriated by the new government (personal communication, Fuad Sirag al-Din).

67. *Al-Ahram,* 5 Apr. 1944.

68. Kirk to Secretary of state, 25 Mar. 1944, RG 84, Box 110, File 812.1, NA.

69. Yusuf, 168–69.

70. Ibid., 170–71; Trefor E. Evans, *The Killearn Diaries, 1934–1946: The Diplomatic and Personal Record of Lord Killearn* (London: Sidgwick and Jackson, 1972), 285–304; Kirk to Secretary of State, 13 Apr. 1944, RG 84, Box 110, File 812.2, NA; Killearn diary, 8, 12, 18 Apr. 1944.

71. Yusuf, 172.
72. Evans, 292.
73. Killearn diary, 21 Apr. 1944.
74. Egypt, *Madhabit,* Senate, sessions of 13 and 24 Apr. 1944, 698–709, 756–63.
75. Ibid., 759.
76. Ibid.
77. Egypt, *Madhabit,* Senate, session of 4 May 1944. The day after Nahhas's speech in the Senate, he had Nagib Mikha'il Bishara, a member of the Kutla party, arrested for distributing pamphlets containing Makram Ebeid's resolutions on the malaria crisis. A few days later Makram Ebeid himself was arrested (Kirk, 12 May 1944, RG 84, Box 110, File 812.2, NA; *Egyptian Gazette,* 10 May 1944).

5. Enter the Rockefeller Foundation

1. *Egyptian Gazette,* 21 Feb. 1944; Soper diary, 24 Feb. 1944; Kerr, *Building the Health Bridge,* 301.
2. Personal communication, Louis A. Riehl.
3. Report on Malaria Control, submitted 28 Mar. 1944, FO 370/927.
4. Killearn diary, 12 Apr. 1944.
5. Personal communication, Muhyi al-Din Farid.
6. Kirk to Secretary of State, 11 Apr. 1944, RG 84, Box 110, file 812.1, NA.
7. Ibid.
8. Killearn to Eden, 22 Apr. 1944, FO 370/927.
9. Memorandum, Rockefeller Foundation, Egypt, 25 Apr. 1944, RG 112, Box 15, file USATC, NA.
10. Killearn to Eden, 22 Apr. 1944, FO 370/927.
11. Ibid.
12. Ibid.
13. Ibid.
14. Personal communication, Muhyi al-Din Farid.
15. Kerr diary, 5 Nov. 1944.
16. The United States had only a legation in Cairo until just after World War II when it became an embassy.
17. Kerr, *Building the Health Bridge,* 301; J. E. Jacobs to Secretary of State, 12 May 1944, RG 84, Box 110, file 812.1, NA.
18. Soper diary, "Notes Taken on Trip to Upper Egypt," 11 May 1944, RG 1.1, Series 485 I, Box 2, Folder 16, RFA; personal communication, Muhyi al-Din Farid.
19. Personal communication, Muhyi al-Din Farid.
20. Soper to Wilson, 2 June 1944, RG 1.1, Series 485, Box 2, RFA.
21. Soper diary, 5 July 1944.
22. Morgan to Rucker, 13 June 1944, FO 371/41372.
23. Killearn diary, 5 June 1944.

24. *Egyptian Gazette,* 18 June 1944.

25. *Journal d'Egypte,* 15 May 1944.

26. DDT is a chemical compound first described by O. Zeigler in 1874 and resynthesized by Paul Müller in Switzerland. Its effectiveness as an insecticide was discovered in New York in the early years of World War II. DDT was widely used by Allied forces when it was believed to be of little danger to human beings and the environment. In 1948 Müller won the Nobel Prize because of the usefulness of DDT in the control of epidemics (K. H. Buechel, ed., *The Chemistry of Pesticides* [New York: Wiley, 1983], 27–28).

27. *Egyptian Gazette,* 1 Aug. 1944.

28. Tuck to Secretary of State, 21 July 1944, RG 84, Box 110, File 812.1, NA.

29. *Egyptian Gazette,* 2 June 1944.

30. Soper diary, 14 July 1944.

31. Ibid.

32. Personal communication, J. Austin Kerr.

33. *Egyptian Gazette,* 11 Aug. 1944; Killearn diary, 13 Aug. 1944.

34. Kerr diary, 16 Sept. 1944

35. Soper diary, 10 July 1944.

36. Kerr, *Building the Health Bridge,* 300.

37. Portuguese is the language spoken in Brazil.

38. Kerr diary, 13 July 1944; Kerr, *Building the Health Bridge,* 301.

39. Soper to Strode, 12 Sept. 1944, RG 1.1, Series 485, Box 2, RFA.

40. Visit of Dr. Pridie to the Gambiae Eradication Service of the Rockefeller Foundation at Asiut: 18–20 Aug., 21 Aug. 1945, FO 370/1107.

41. Preliminary Survey of the Medical Services of Egypt, 24 Aug. 1945, FO 371/45990.

42. Kerr diary, 12 Sept. 1944.

43. *Egyptian Gazette,* 11 Sept. 1944.

44. Kerr diary, 10 Oct. 1944.

45. Yusuf, 190.

46. Kerr diary, 10 Oct. 1944.

47. *Egyptian Mail,* 31 Oct. 1944.

48. *Egyptian Gazette,* 25 Oct. 1944.

49. Kerr to Strode, 14 Nov. 1944, RG 1.1, Series 485, Box 2, RA.

50. *Plasmodium vivax* as opposed to *Plasmodium falciparum.*

51. Al-Ahram, 3 Nov. 1944.

52. Kerr diary, 23 Nov. 1944 and 25 Jan. 1945; Kerr to Strode, 14 Nov. 1944, RG 1.1, Series 485, Box 2, RFA.

53. Kerr, *Building the Health Bridge,* 301.

54. Kerr diary, 6 Nov. 1944.

55. Ibid., 4 Nov. 1944.

56. Ibid., 6 Nov. 1944.

57. Ibid., 12 Nov. 1944.

58. Ibid., 5 Dec. 1944.

59. Ibid.

60. Ibid., 13 Jan. 1945.

61. Ibid., 11 Feb. 1945.

62. Ibid., 24 Mar. 1945.

63. Egypt, *Annual Report* (1944), 85.

64. Ibid., 88. The Ministry of Health states, "A new chapter in the use of D.D.T. was started in November 1944, when the ceilings of railway coaches were spray-painted with a 10% D.D.T. and kerosene solution. This was perhaps the first time this method was practised in the whole world." See also Egypt, *Annual Report* (1945), 93.

65. Egypt, *Annual Report* (1944), 89.

66. Egypt, *Annual Report* (1945), 91.

67. Kerr, *Building the Health Bridge*, 301.

68. For a description of the final stages of the eradication process, see Egypt, *Annual Report* (1945), 95.

69. Kerr diary, 7 Nov. 1944.

70. *Egyptian Gazette,* 5 Jan. 1945; Kerr diary, 5 Jan. 1945.

71. *Akhbar al-Yawm,* 10 Oct. 1945; Kerr diary, 10 Oct. 1945.

72. Kerr diary, 2 Dec. 1945; personal communication, Muhyi al-Din Farid.

73. Egypt, *Annual Report* (1945), 97.

74. Soper diary, 4 Jan. 1946; Kerr diary, 4 Jan. 1946.

75. *Al-Ahram,* 5 Jan. 1946.

76. Kerr diary, 4 Jan. 1946.

77. John M. Weir, "Report on the Medical Services and Public Health Facilities of Egypt," Rockefeller Foundation Archives, RG 1.2, 485 J, 30.

78. Egypt, *Annual Report* (1945), 93, 97. In 1950, when *A. gambiae* mosquitoes again appeared inside Egypt at Abu Simbil, staff members from the Malaria Section and the Insect Eradication Section immediately exterminated them (A. Halawani and A. A. Shawarby, "Malaria in Egypt [History, Epidemiology, Control and Treatment]," *Egyptian Medical Association Journal* 40, no. 11 [1957]: 778–79; Shawarby et al., 194–95. For more recent control measures see G. R. Shidrawi, "Report on a Mission to Upper Egypt and Sudan in Connection with *A. Gambiae* (Arabiensis) Protective and Control Measures," Unpublished Paper (Cairo: World Health Organization, July 1980).

79. Health workers have subsequently learned that malaria control is a political and social problem requiring much longer than five years. Many strains of mosquito are resistant to DDT and its derivatives, and malaria is more widespread in Central America and sub-Saharan Africa and elsewhere than it was in Brazil and Egypt. Researchers are currently attempting to develop a vaccine against malaria.

80. Egypt, *Taqrir al-jambiyya,* 2.

81. Soper diary, 14 July 1944.

6. *British-American Rivalries*

1. John A. DeNovo, "The Culbertson Economic Mission and Anglo-American Tensions in the Middle East, 1944–1945," *Journal of American History*

63 (Dec.–Mar. 1976–77): 913–36; Elizabeth Monroe, *Britain's Moment in the Middle East, 1914–1971* (London: Chatto and Windus, 1981), 161–62.

2. Killearn to Eden, 9 May 1944, FO 371/41372.

3. Confidential note regarding the necessity of a British medical research institute, 9 May 1944, FO 371/41372.

4. Ibid.

5. Ibid.

6. Ibid.

7. Ibid.

8. The Wellcome Trust was set up in London in 1936 from the estate of Sir Henry Solomon Wellcome, the pharmaceutical manufacturer, primarily for the support of medical research. For information in its early years see *Report— Wellcome Trust, 1937–1956* (London: The Wellcome Trust, 1957). For a favorable response to a medical research station in Egypt, see M. T. Morgan: "Research Center in Egypt," 22 June 1944, FO 371/41372.

9. Killearn to Eden, 27 June 1944, FO 371/41372.

10. Killearn diary, 18 Apr. 1945.

11. Killearn to Eden, 20 July 1945, FO 371/1107.

12. Louis, *British Empire in the Middle East,* vii–viii; Monroe, 160–61.

13. For earlier examples of the politics of quarantining, see Goodman, 60–61.

14. Kerr diary, 12 Dec. 1944; Egypt, *Madhabit,* Senate, 15 Dec. 1947.

15. Telegram, Killearn to Foreign Office, 31 Aug. 1942, FO 371/35598.

16. Memorandum, 6 Oct. 1944, FO 371/41366.

17. One British official remained attached to the quarantine service in Alexandria until 1945 (Preliminary Survey of the Medical Services of Egypt, 24 Aug. 1945, FO 371/45990).

18. Killearn to Eden, 9 May 1944, FO 371/41372.

19. Review by E. D. Pridie, Oct. 1945, FO 371/45991; Pridie's duties, 18 May 1946, FO 371/53279; Note by E. D. Pridie, 29 Apr. 1946, FO 371/53279.

20. Memorandum from Pridie, 8 Aug. 1945, FO 371/45990.

21. Ibid.

22. Preliminary Survey of the Medical Services of Egypt, 24 Aug. 1945, FO 371/45990.

23. Ibid.

24. Ibid.

25. DeNovo, "Culbertson Economic Mission," 933–35.

26. Kerr diary, 5 and 15 Jan. 1945.

27. Soper diary, 4 Jan. 1946.

28. Kerr diary, 20 June 1945.

29. Ibid., 27 July 1945.

30. NAMRU-1 was at the University of California, Berkeley, from 1944 to 1974. NAMRU-2 was commissioned in New York in 1944 and was immediately moved to the Pacific. After the war it was closed for a few years; in 1957 it was reestablished in Taipei. NAMRU-3 has functioned from 1945 to the present in Egypt. NAMRU-4 was in the Great Lakes Training Center from 1948 to 1974.

NAMRU-5 was established in Ethiopia from 1965 to 1978. The units study diseases likely to endanger American troops. van Heyningen and Seal, 68–70.

31. *La bourse egyptienne,* 13 Nov. 1945.

32. Ibid.

33. Ahmad Mahir, the prime minister, had been walking to Parliament to declare war symbolically on the side of Britain against Germany when an anti-British nationalist had assassinated him in February 1945, whereupon Mahmud Fahmi al-Nuqrashi became prime minister.

34. *Egyptian Mail,* 6 Dec. 1945.

35. Waring to Bayne-Jones, 7 Dec. 1945, RG 112, Box 57 (R), USATC, NA.

36. *New York Times,* 2 Mar. 1946.

37. R. A. Graff to Sheldon Dudley, 12 Oct. 1945, FO 371/45991.

38. "Visit paid by Dr. Pridie to the Abbasiyya infectious diseases hospital," 22 Oct. 1945, FO 371/45991.

39. Minute by Dr. Pridie, 22 Nov. 1945, FO 371/45991.

40. Ibid.

41. Ibid.

42. Ibid.

43. Telegram, FO to Cairo, for Pridie, 4 May 1946, FO 371/53278.

44. Report on a Visit by Dr. Pridie to Dr. Shusha Pasha, Undersecretary of State for Medical Affairs at the Ministry of Public Health, 5 Jan. 1946, FO 371/45991.

45. Killearn to Bevin, 26 Nov. 1945, FO 371/45991.

46. Ibid.

47. Yates to Lambert, 15 Dec. 1945, FO 371/45991.

48. Egyptian Department to Chancery, British Embassy Washington, D.C., 5 Jan. 1946, FO 371/45991; Michael Wright to P. S. Scrivener, Jan. 1946, FO 371/53277.

49. Killearn to R. G. Howe, 14 Jan. 1946, FO 371/53278; Note by E. D. Pridie, 29 Apr. 1946, FO 371/53279.

50. Louis, *British Empire in the Middle East,* 15–21.

51. Kerr diary, 19 Feb. 1946; Tariq al-Bishri, *al-Harakat al-siyasiyya fi misr, 1945–1952* (The Political Movement in Egypt, 1945–1952), 2d ed. (Beirut: Dar al-Shuruq, 1983), 205–6.

52. *Egyptian Gazette,* 17 Mar. 1946.

53. Ahmed Hussein, *Rural Social Welfare Centres in Egypt* (Cairo: Ministry of Social Affairs, 1951), 5.

54. *Al-Ahram,* 15 Nov. 1946.

55. Report by Dr. Pridie, 12 Mar. 1946, FO 371/53278; Note on Health Centres, 5 Apr. 1946, FO 371/53279.

56. Visit with Azmi Pasha, 6 Mar. 1946, FO 371/53278.

57. Interview with Sidqi, 12 Mar. 1946, FO 371/53728.

58. Ibid.

59. Kerr diary, 6 Dec. 1945.

60. Wilson to Strode, 18 June 1946, RG 1.1, Series 485, Box 2, RFA.

61. Kerr diary, 18 Oct. 1945.

62. Ibid., 19 Feb. 1946.

63. Ibid.

64. M. Gaud, Muhammad Khalil (Abd al-Khaliq), and M. Vaucel, "The Evolution of the Epidemic of Relapsing Fever, 1942–1946," *Bulletin of the World Health Organization* 1, no. 2 (1948): 93–101.

65. Following an outbreak of relapsing fever in 1926, there had been one reported case of this disease in 1932, one in 1933, three in 1934, two in 1936, and one in 1940 (Egypt, *Annual Report* [1945], 9).

66. Ibid.

67. Ibid.

68. Memorandum of Conversation between Radi Bey, Undersecretary of the Ministry of Social Affairs and William J. Handley, 3 Apr. 1946, RG 59, File 883, NA.

69. Appendix B (translation of *Journal d'Egypte*, 1 Apr. 1947), attached to Memorandum regarding the higher council of ministers set up by the Egyptian government to deal with poverty, ignorance, and disease, 12 Apr. 1946, FO 371/53279; *al-Ahram*, 1 Apr. 1946.

70. The Muslim Brotherhood (Ikhwan al-Muslimin) had been formed by Hasan al-Banna in 1928 or 1929. Members believed that only a return to Islamic principles could set Egypt on the road to progress. The organization advocated social, economic, and public health reform and nationalization of foreign companies. To this end it published its own newspaper, weekly magazine, and other publications, all of which enjoyed a wide circulation in the postwar era. The organization, which at times enjoyed good relations with the palace, became increasingly militant in the 1940s, when it was implicated in a series of assassinations and bombings.

71. Richard P. Mitchell, *The Society of the Muslim Brothers* (London: Oxford Univ. Press, 1969), 289–94.

72. An extended study of the activities of the Muslim Brotherhood and the other Islamic groups in public health and medicine is much needed.

73. *Al-Nadhir*, 45 (June 1946).

74. Ibid.

75. *Al-Ahram*, 19 Mar. 1946.

76. Ibid., 2 and 5 Apr. 1946.

77. Ibid., 25 Mar. 1946.

78. Waring to Bayne-Jones, 11 Feb. 1946, RG 112, Box 57(R), USATC, NA.

79. *Washington Post*, 29 Mar. 1946; Kerr diary, 29 Mar. 1946.

80. Kerr diary, 4 Apr. 1946; *al-Ahram*, 5 Apr. 1946.

81. Ahmed Hussein, *Social Welfare*, 29.

82. Egypt, *Annual Report* (1946), 9.

83. Egypt, *Annual Report* (1947), 15. The report gives 10 officially reported cases during 1944; 18,126 during 1945; and 110,405 during 1946. A. M. Kamal (*Epidemiology of Communicable Diseases* [Cairo: Anglo-American Bookshop,

1958] 223) gives 10 officially recorded cases in 1944; 18,477 in 1945; and 108,882 in 1946, for a total of 127,369 cases.

84. Egypt, *Annual Report* (1947), 15. The report lists no deaths in 1944; 881 deaths in 1945; 2,414 in 1946; and 30 in 1947. Report on relapsing fever, 14 May 1946, FO 371/53278.

85. Khalil, "The 1936 Treaty," 5.

86. Kamal, 217–26.

87. Evans, 372.

7. Cholera Goes out of Control

1. *Akhbar al-Yawm,* 27 Sept. 1947.

2. *Al-Ahram,* 24 Sept. 1947; *al-Balagh,* 24 Sept. 1947.

3. *Aklhbar al-Yawm,* 27 Sept. 1947.

4. *Kashkul,* 27 Sept. 1947.

5. *Al-Balagh,* 27 Sept. 1947.

6. *Akhbar al-Yawm,* 4 Oct. 1947.

7. Robert L. Buell to Secretary of State, 25 Sept. 1947, RG 59, File 158.832/9-2547, NA.

8. Ayrout, 79–80.

9. *Akhir Saʿa,* 1 Oct. 1947.

10. *Akhbar al-Yawm,* 27 Sept. 1947.

11. Wilson was the former field director of the Gambiae Eradication Service and at the time field staff director of the Africa and Asia Minor Region of the International Health Division of the Rockefeller Foundation.

12. Wilson to Strode, 30 Sept. 1947, RG 2, Series 485, Box 385, Folder 2600, RFA.

13. *Ruz al-Yusuf,* 1 Oct. 1947.

14. *Ruz al-Yusuf,* 1 Oct. 1947.

15. Villages served by rural social centers and health units had low rates of infection (Ahmed Hussein, *Social Welfare,* 29).

16. Ahmed Hussein, *Social Welfare,* 76.

17. Wilson to Strode, 4 Oct. 1947, No. 21–47, RG 2, Series 485, Box 385, Folder 2600, RFA.

18. *Akhir Saʿa,* 15 Oct. 1947.

19. *Al-Balagh,* 20 Oct. 1947.

20. *Al-Musawwar,* 3 Oct. 1947.

21. *Egyptian Gazette,* 22 Oct. 1947.

22. Andree Chedid, The Sixth Day (London: A. Blond, 1962).

23. Ibid., 12–14. Yusuf Chahine, the noted Egyptian film producer, has adapted the book for a film of the same name (*Yawm al-Sadis,* 1986).

24. Weekly Appreciation, Campbell to Bevin, 1 Nov. 1947, FO 371/63021.

25. *Egyptian Gazette,* 28 Oct. 1947.

26. *Akhir Saʿa,* 12 Nov. 1947.

27. *Ikhwan al-Muslimin* (daily), 30 Sept. 1947.

28. *Ikhwan al-Muslimin* (weekly), 18 Oct. 1947.

29. Young Egypt (Misr al-Fatat) was founded by Ahmad Husayn as a movement in 1933 and as a formal political party in January 1937. It was a nationalist party that patterned itself after the fascist organizations of Europe. Husayn believed that poverty was caused by the British, who had not encouraged industry or sufficient land reclamation to support Egypt's growing population.

30. *Misr al-Fatat,* 29 Sept. 1947.

31. Ibid., 20 Oct. 1947.

32. Ibid., 27 Oct. 1947.

33. Ibid., 20 Oct. 1947.

34. *Kutla,* 30 Sept. 1947.

35. *Al-Balagh,* 27 Sept. 1947.

36. Weekly Appreciation, 8 Nov. 1947, FO 371/63021.

37. *Al-Balagh,* 30 Oct. 1947.

38. Ibid.

39. A few small, disunited communist groups had been formed in the 1930s. Their members, who were largely drawn from minority groups within Egypt, were initially motivated by the struggle against fascism. In the 1940s the communist groups worked toward workers' rights and international socialist revolution. The groups were small in number and in membership but very influential in the labor movement, which became increasingly militant in the postwar era. In May 1947 two of the larger groups united and formed the Democratic Movement for National Liberation (al-Harakat al-dimuqratiyya lil-tahrir al-watani) or Haditu, the acronym for the Arabic name. Haditu quickly became the major communist party of Egypt. It took over publication of the weekly newspaper, *al-Jamahir* (*The Masses*), which had been founded the previous month.

40. *Al-Jamahir,* 19 and 26 Oct. 1947.

41. Ibid., 12 Oct. 1947.

42. Ibid., 5 Oct. 1947.

43. Ibid., 19 Oct. 1947.

44. van Heyningen and Seal, 68–74.

45. *United States Information Service Bulletin,* Cairo, 27–28 Sept. 1947.

46. Robert L. Buell to S. Pinkney Tuck, 1 Oct. 1947, RG 84, Box 171, File 812.1, NA.

47. William L. Jenkins to S. Pinkney Tuck, 4 Nov. 1947, RG 59, File 883.00/ 11-447, NA.

48. *Le Phare egyptien,* 7 Oct. 1947.

49. Gillespie S. Evans to Hilton W. Rose, 20 Oct. 1947, RG 84, Box 171, File 812.1, NA.

50. Emile T. Rumpp to Mrs. Harry K. [*sic*] Truman, 4 Oct. 1947, enclosing translation of article in *Journal d'Egypte,* 30 Sept. 1947, RG 84, Box 171, File 812.1, NA.

51. *Egyptian Mail,* 29 and 30 Sept. 1947.

52. United Kingdom, Hansard (P. Ford and G. Ford), *Catalogue Breviate of Parliamentary Papers* 443 (Oxford, 1961), 5 Nov. 1947, col. 1817.

53. Request for ambulances, 24 Oct. 1947, FO 371/63111.

54. United Kingdom, *House of Commons Parliamentary Papers* 444, col. 369; *Egyptian Gazette*, 16 Nov. 1947.

55. Pridie papers, 27–28.

56. *Yearbook of the United Nations*, 1947–48, 916.

57. Memo on Tass communiqué, 6 Oct. 1947, RG 59, File 158.832/10-647.

58. *Al-Musawwar*, 31 Oct. 1947.

59. *Al-Ahram*, 12 Oct. 1947; *New York Times*, 18 Oct. 1947.

60. *Al-Ahram*, 12 Oct. 1947.

61. Ibid., 29 Sept. 1947.

62. *New York Times*, 30 Oct. 1947.

63. Ibid., 29 Oct. 1947; *Akhbar al-Yawm*, 1 Nov. 1947.

64. United States Information Service Bulletin: "Ministry of Public Health Thanks Legation of China for Largest Vaccine Gift," 4 Nov. 1947; Memorandum, G. S. Evans to William K. McNown, 7 Nov. 1947, RG 84, Box 171, File 812.1, NA.

65. Bruce White, "Report on a Visit to Cairo Made on Behalf of the Medical Research Council and Ministry of Health with Notes on Some Laboratory Studies Made in Connection with the 1947 Autumn Epidemic of Cholera in Egypt." Unpublished manuscript. Archives of the Medical Research Council, Mill Hill, London, 1947.

66. *Al-Assas*, 5 Nov. 1947.

67. Wilson to Strode, 11 Oct. 1947, RG 2, Series 485, Box 385, Folder 2600, RFA.

68. Ibid.

69. Wilson to Strode, 1 Oct. 1947, RG 2, Series 485, RFA.

70. Personal communication, Adil Sabit.

71. "General Report of the Functions of the Anti-Fly Campaign Committee formed by the Ministry of Health of the Egyptian Government in Connection with the Problem of Fly Control during the Cholera Epidemic of 1947," Ministry of Public Health, Egypt, n.d.; *London Times*, 5 Oct. 1947; Wilson to Strode, 18 Oct. 1947, RG 2, Series 485, RFA.

72. Wilson to Strode, 11 Oct. 1947, RG 2, Series 485, RFA.

73. Tuck to Secretary of State, 30 Oct. 1947, RG 59, File 158.832/10-3047, NA.

74. Ali Tawfiq Shusha, "Cholera Epidemic in Egypt (1947): A Preliminary Report," *Bulletin of the World Health Organization* 1, no. 2 (1948): 368–69.

75. *Official Record of the World Health Organization* 8 (1948): 27–28.

76. *Al-Musawwar*, 30 Oct. 1947.

77. Ibid., 24 Oct. 1947; *London Times*, 31 Oct. 1947; Decree of the Ministry of Public Health, 3 Nov. 1947, RG 59, File 883.00/10-1047, NA.

78. *Al-Ahram*, 25 Sept. 1947; Shusha, "Cholera Epidemic," 357–62.

79. Weekly Appreciation, 8 Nov. 1947, FO 371/63071.

80. *Egyptian Gazette*, 14 Oct. 1947.

81. *Al-Misri,* 19 Oct. 1947; *al-Balagh,* 30 Oct. 1947.

82. *Al-Kutla,* 30 Sept. 1947.

83. *Ithnayn wa Dunya,* 6 Oct. 1947.

84. *Akhir Sa'a,* 1 Oct. 1947; *Akhbar,* 1 Nov. 1947; *al-Ahram,* 30 Oct. 1947.

85. Berque, 614.

86. The *zakat* is usually about 2.5 percent for Muslims. *Akhir Sa'a,* 22 Oct. 1947.

87. *Kashkul,* 3 Nov. 1947.

88. *Al-Ahram,* 3 Nov. 1947.

89. Weekly Appreciation, 8 Nov. 1947, FO 371/63021.

90. *Al-Ahram,* 30 Oct. 1947.

91. Hussein, *Social Welfare,* 74.

92. *Al-Musawwar,* 7 Nov. 1947.

93. Ibid., 31 Oct. 1947; *al-Ahram,* 3 Nov. 1947.

94. *Egyptian Gazette,* 11 and 24 Nov. 1947.

95. Hussein, *Social Welfare,* 76.

96. Egypt, *Annual Report* (1947), 15.

97. Decree proclaiming Egypt free of cholera epidemic, 11 Feb. 1948, RG 59, File No. 158.832/1-2748, NA.

98. *Yearbook of the United Nations,* 1947–48, 916; and Goodman, 173.

99. Kamal, 159; Zaghloul, 218.

100. Kamal, 138–63.

101. "Award of the Shusha Prize," *Journal of the Egyptian Public Health Association* 43, no. 5 (1968): 425.

102. Weir to Strode, 25 Nov. 1947, RG 2, Series 485, Box 385, Folder 2600, RFA.

103. Wilson to Strode, 12 Dec. 1947, RG 2, Series 485, Box 385, Folder 2600, RFA.

104. A. H. Kurdi (A. H. Kordi), "Some Observations on the Effect of Cholera Vaccine during the Recent Cholera Epidemic in Egypt," *Journal of the Royal Egyptian Medical Association* 31, no. 4 (Apr. 1948): 289–99.

105. *World Health Organization Epidemiological and Vital Statistics Report,* Dec. 1947, 72–74, 149; Ali H. al-Ramli, "Clinical Study of 689 Cases of Cholera Isolated in the Abbassia Fever Hospital," *Journal of the Royal Egyptian Medical Association* 31, no. 4 (Apr. 1948): 322–50.

106. General Political Review of 1947, FO 371/73458.

107. Memoir of Sir Eric Denholm Pridie, Oriental Section, University Library, Durham University.

108. Abd al-Rahman al-Raf'i, *Fi aqab al-thawrat al-misryya* (The Consequences of the Egyptian Revolution) (Cairo: Maktabat al-nahda al-misriyya, 1951), 3: 255.

8. The British Connection

1. *Egyptian Gazette,* 8 and 22 Sept. 1947; *al-Balagh,* 22 Sept. 1947.

2. Louis, *British Empire in the Middle East,* 9–10.

3. Muhammed Hasanayn Haykal (Mohamed Heikal), *The Cairo Documents: The Inside Story of Nasser and His Relationship with World Leaders, Rebels, and Statesmen* (New York: Doubleday, 1973), xvii.

4. *Akhbar al-Yawm,* 27 Sept. 1947 and 4 Oct. 1947.

5. Ibid., 25 Oct. 1947.

6. Ibid., 11 Nov. 1947.

7. *Al-Misri,* quoted in *Egyptian Gazette,* 26 Sept. 1947.

8. *Al-Balagh,* 27 Sept. 1947.

9. Ibid., 7 and 9 Oct. 1947.

10. *Ikhwan al-Muslimin* (weekly), 4 Oct. 1947.

11. *Ikhwan al-Muslimin* (daily), 24 Sept. 1947.

12. Ibid., 2 Oct. 1947.

13. *Ikhwan al-Muslimin* (weekly), 4 Oct. 1947.

14. Ibid., 4 Oct. 1947.

15. *Ikhwan al-Muslimin* (daily), quoted in *Egyptian Gazette,* 7 Oct. 1947.

16. *Ikhwan al-Muslimin* (weekly), 4 Oct. 1947.

17. *Minbar al-sharq,* quoted in *Egyptian Gazette,* 13 Oct. 1947.

18. *Al-Ikhwan al-Muslimin* (weekly), 25 Oct. 1947.

19. *Al-Jamahir,* 28 Sept. 1947.

20. Ibid., 5 Oct. 1947.

21. Ibid.

22. The British embassy reported, "a report from a secret source states that a pamphlet has been circulated by the Egyptian communist organization, Hameto-Shar, giving its members guidance in the exploitation of the cholera epidemic for political purposes" (Weekly Appreciation, 8 Nov. 1947, FO 371/63021).

23. Weekly Appreciation, 28 Oct. 1947, FO 371/63021.

24. *Misr al-Fatat,* 6 and 20 Oct. 1947.

25. *Egyptian Gazette,* 25 Sept. 1947.

26. Ibid., 6 Oct. 1947.

27. Weekly Appreciation, 11 Oct. 1947, FO 371/63021.

28. Ibid., 3 Oct. 1947.

29. According to the British embassy, Huda Sha'rawi was "violently anti-British and on behalf of the Egyptian Feminist Movement frequently sent protests to this Embassy, the last occasion being on the subject of Palestine only a few days before her death" (Weekly Appreciation, 20 Dec. 1947, FO 371/63021). She died on 12 December 1947.

30. *Egyptian Gazette,* 13 Nov. 1947.

31. United Kingdom, Hansard (P. Ford and G. Ford), *Catalogue Breviate of Parliamentary Papers* (Oxford, 1961), 444, no. 12 (Nov. 1947–48), col. 368.

32. Ibid., cols. 368–69.

33. *Egyptian Gazette,* 7 Nov. 1947.

34. Ibid., 11 and 14 Nov. 1947.

35. *The Lancet,* 11 Oct. 1947, 551.

36. Ibid., 25 Oct. 1947, 636.

37. Ibid.

38. Ibid., 1 Nov. 1947, 657.

39. *Egyptian Gazette*, 21 Nov. 1947.

40. *The Lancet*, 8 Nov. 1947.

41. Khalil, "The 1936 Treaty," 9–10. Khalil Abd al-Khaliq also included outbreaks of plague and typhus in his paper on the relationship between war and disease. From 1943 to 1947 the Ministry of Health recorded 1,229 cases of plague and 676 deaths from plague, which Khalil Abd al-Khaliq ascribed to the British Military authorities' having failed to observe quarantine measures at Suez and Port Said. Incidence of typhus, an endemic disease in Egypt, also increased owing to overcrowding, lack of cleanliness, and undernourishment. The ministry's disinfection procedures helped control the disease, and recorded deaths averaged about four thousand per year from 1941 to 1945 (Khalil, "The 1936 Treaty," 5–6). As mentioned above, typhus did not have a great political impact because it was a very common disease in Egypt and therefore lacked the "shock value" of malignant malaria, relapsing fever, and cholera.

42. Khalil, "Absolute Humidity," 68.

43. Egypt, *Madhabit*, Senate, session of 15 Dec. 1947, 106–7.

44. The first assembly of the World Health Organization met in Geneva in 1948.

45. Aviation-quarantine, 14 May 1947, FO 141/975.

46. Note on the Pan-Arab Health Bureau, 13 June 1947, FO 957/6.

47. Ibid.

48. Khalil, "Defence of Egypt," 634.

49. Ibid., 636.

50. Khalil, "Absolute Humidity," 69–72; *Akhir Saʿa*, 22 Oct. 1947; *Akhbar al-Yawm*, 8 Nov. 1947.

51. Khalil, "Absolute Humidity," 18.

52. *Akhbar al-Yawm*, 8 Nov. 1947; Saʿid Abduh, "Wabaʾ al-kulira al-hali: kayf nashaʾ wa kayf intashar" (The Current Cholera Epidemic: How it Originated and How it Spread), *Journal of the Royal Egyptian Medical Association* 30, no. 11 (Nov. 1947): 480–99.

53. *Al-Ahram*, 7 Oct. 1947.

54. Shusha, "Cholera Epidemic," 353–81.

55. *Official Record of the World Health Organization* 8 (1948): 27–28.

56. *Al-Assas*, 2 and 14 Nov. 1947.

57. Ibid., 24 Dec. 1947.

58. Egypt, *Annual Report* (1947), 15.

59. Kamal, 152–55.

60. Personal communication, Salah Atiyya.

61. Wilson to Strode, 18 Oct. 1947, attachment, RG 2, Series 485, Box 385, Folder 2600, RFA; personal communication, Abd al-Aziz Salah.

62. Egypt, *Madhabit*, Senate, session of 15 Dec. 1947, 104–5.

63. Ibid., 110.

64. Ibid., 105.

65. Ibid., 115.
66. Ibid., 115–20 and session of 16 Dec. 1947, 120–32.
67. Egypt, *Madhabit,* Chamber of Deputies, sessions of 15–16, 22, and 27 Dec. 1947, and 13 Jan. 1948.
68. Egypt, *Madhabit,* Chamber of Deputies, session of 22 Dec. 1947.
69. Yves Biraud and P. M. Kaul, *World Health Organization Epidemiological and Vital Statistics Report* (Dec. 1947), 152.
70. *Al-Ahram,* 4 Dec. 1947.
71. The missing files contained about thirty documents. For the complete list of document titles see the *Foreign Office Index* (1947), 685–86; (1949), 703.
72. Goodman, 226.
73. "History of Cholera in Egypt" (editorial), *British Medical Journal* 1, no. 1 (Mar. 1951): 688.
74. Taha Husayn, *al-Mu'adhdhabun fi al-'ardh* (The Wretched of the Earth) (Cairo: al-Kitab al-fiddiy, 1958), 182–92. Publication of the book, which was completed in 1948, was initially forbidden in Egypt, so the author had it published first in Lebanon and much later in Cairo. In the chapter entitled "al-Mu'tazila" (The Withdrawn One [fem.]), the author relates the tragic story of Um Tammam, her son, and of her daughter in a village in Upper Egypt during the 1902 cholera epidemic. The son died of cholera. The despondent mother tried to drown herself and her daughter. The mother died but the daughter was pulled from the canal alive. She lived but became insane, sitting endlessly beside the canal. Taha Husayn concluded that, while social and political conditions in Egypt had changed between 1902 and 1947, the disease could still go from village to village and that nothing prevented such events from recurring.

9. Public Health on the National Agenda

1. Quoted in Ayrout, 74–75. The book was first published in French in 1938, in English in 1945, and revised for republication in 1963.
2. Ibid.
3. Ahmed Hussein, *Social Welfare,* 129.
4. Facilities were reopened in 1953 after the revolution, but in January 1954 they were taken over by the government (Mitchell, 290).
5. *Al-Musawwar,* translated and paraphrased in Jefferson Patterson to Secretary of State, 14 Mar. 1949, RG 59, File 883.00/3-1449, NA.
6. *Akhir Sa'a,* translated and paraphrased in Jefferson Patterson to Secretary of State, 14 Mar. 1949, RG 59, File 883.00/3-1449, NA.
7. *Akhir Sa'a,* 14 Nov. 1949.
8. Withdrawal of Misr al Fattat from Support of Present Government, 12 July 1949, RG 59, File 883.00/7-1249, NA.
9. Editorials on Social Justice and the Fellah in *Al Misri,* 12 May 1949, RG 59, File 883.00/5-1249; Arabic Press Review, *Egyptian Gazette,* 10 May 1949.
10. *Egyptian Gazette,* 20 Apr. 1949.

11. Weekly Appreciation, 19 Apr. 1947, FO 371/63020; *Egyptian Gazette,* 23 Apr. 1947; *al-Ahram,* 2 May 1947; *Egyptian Gazette,* 1 June 1944.

12. Egyptian Water Purification Scheme, Campbell to Bevin, 17 Dec. 1947, FO 371/63115.

13. Ibid.

14. Personal communication, Abd al-Aziz Salah.

15. General Political Review of 1947, FO 371/73458.

16. Plan for social reform in Egypt, 15 Feb. 1948, FO 371/69230.

17. Campbell to FO, Report by Mr. W. J. Johnson on the Egyptian financial and economic situation, 16 May 1949, FO 371/73515.

18. A. A. F. Haigh to Establishment and Finance Department, 28 Jan. 1948, FO 371/69230.

19. John M. Weir, "Report on the Medical Services and Public Health Facilities of Egypt," Rockefeller Foundation Archives, RG 1.2, 485 J, 30.

20. Ibid., 34–36.

21. Ibid., 96.

22. Ibid., 108.

23. Ibid., 112.

24. U.S. Government Official Text, Addresses delivered 27 Oct. 1947, issued by U.S. Information Service, n.d., NAMRU-3 Archives.

25. *Al-Misri,* 25 Feb. 1948, translated in NAMRU-3 Archives.

26. Ibid.

27. *Al-Kutla,* 17 Feb. 1948, translated in NAMRU-3 Archives.

28. *Al-Musawwar,* 19 Feb. 1948, translated in NAMRU-3 Archives.

29. Official Text, 27 Oct. 1947; *Al-Ahram,* 28 Oct. 1948.

30. Official Text, 27 Oct. 1947.

31. Ibid.

32. *Al-Siyasa,* 28 Oct. 1948.

33. For a discussion of this Wafdist government's political difficulties see Joel Gordon, "The False Hopes of 1950: The Wafd's Last Hurrah and the Demise of Egypt's Old Order," *International Journal of Middle East Studies* 21, no. 2 (May 1989): 193–214.

34. Editorials on Social Justice and the Fellah in *Al Misri,* 12 May 1949, RG 59, File 883.00/5-1249; Tom Little, *Modern Egypt* (New York: Ernest Benn, 1967), 105.

35. For an optimistic account of these reforms, see Ahmed Hussein, *Social Welfare,* 109–18.

36. Al-Bishri, *al-Harakat,* 228–29.

37. Gamal Abdul Nasser, *Egypt's Liberation: The Philosophy of the Revolution* (Washington, D.C.: Public Affairs Press, 1955), 39–40.

38. *The Egyptian Gazette,* 9 June 1953, quoted in H. Jackson Davis, "A Health and Sanitation Program in Egypt," 4 July 1953, NA 59 A–758, Box 60.

39. Ministry of Health, Arab Republic of Egypt, *Egyptian Experience in Primary Health Care,* n.d., 13; Ahmed Hussein, *Rural Social Welfare Centres,* 5; Ahmed Hussein, *Social Welfare,* 15.

40. James B. Mayfield, *Rural Politics in Nasser's Egypt: A Quest for Legitimacy* (Austin: Univ. of Texas Press, 1971), 181.

41. Raymond Baker, *Egypt's Uncertain Revolution under Nasser and Sadat* (Cambridge, Mass.: Harvard Univ. Press, 1978), 218.

42. A good description of a rural health center is provided by Ayrout, 77–78.

43. A. K. Mazen, "Development of the Medical Care Program of the Egyptian Region of the United Arab Republic" (Ph.D. diss., Stanford Univ., 1961), 50.

44. On 11 February 1949 (the king's birthday), the Mabarra had, for example, established a clinic in Port Said to serve the poor and indigent. A month later Princess Fawziyya presided over the laying of the cornerstone for its permanent buildings. The clinic reported serving 158,230 patients from February to December 1948 ("Official Opening of the Clinic and Dispensary 'Oeuvre Mohamed Aly El-Kebir,'" 19 Mar. 1949, RG 59, File 883.247, NA).

45. Istiphan, 145–46.

46. Ibid., 211–12. The Egyptian Red Crescent Association, headed by Sulayman Azmi, listed thirty-three volunteers. It reported that the Red Crescent had served "12,000 individuals of all religions and nationalities, of all ages and both sexes" (Istiphan, 67–68).

47. Ahmed Hussein, *Social Welfare,* 91–108.

48. Law No. 384 of 1956 is published in Istiphan, Appendix IV.

49. Mazen, 76–77.

50. Ibid., 31.

51. George Rosen, *A History of Public Health* (New York: M. D. Publications, 1958), 485.

52. H. Jackson Davis, "A Health and Sanitation Program in Egypt," 4 July 1953, NA USOM/E, 59A-758, Box 60.

53. Ibid., 27.

54. Hrair Dekmajian, "An Analytical History and Evaluation of the Egyptian-American Rural Improvement Service (EARIS), 1953–1965." Unpublished paper (Washington, D.C.: U.S. Agency for International Development [Apr. 1981]), 21.

55. NA USOM/E Public Health Files, 1953–54, 59A-758, Box 58.

56. NAMRU-3 remained in operation during the Suez Crisis of 1956 and during the 1967 Six-Day War when the American staff was forced to leave Egypt for a few days.

57. Quoted in Baker, 218.

58. Mayfield, 180–86; Baker, 224–32.

59. Baker, 220–21.

60. Mayfield, 185.

61. Baker, 231–32.

62. Ibid., 228.

63. Mayfield, 186, 207–10.

64. Baker, 224–25ff.

65. A. A. Afifi and L. A. Sagan, "Energy and Literacy: An Index of Health Development." Unpublished Paper (Vienna: International Institute for Applied Systems Analysis, Aug. 1978), 14–15.

66. Those who survived their first year lived an average of nine years longer. Ministry of Health, Arab Republic of Egypt: *Basic Statistical Information on Health Services,* Cairo (July 1977), 3, cited in "Health in Egypt: Recommendations for U.S. Assistance" (Washington, D.C.: Institute of Medicine, Jan. 1979), 39.

Bibliography

Government and Private Archives

Archives of the United States Naval Research Unit, Number 3 (NAMRU-3), Cairo, Egypt.
Rockefeller Foundation Archives, Tarrytown, N.Y. (RFA)
    RG 1.1, Series 485.
United Kingdom. Public Record Office
    FO 141 (Embassy and Consular Archives, Egypt—Correspondence).
    FO 370 (General Correspondence, Library).
    FO 371 (Foreign Office, Political—Egypt and Sudan).
    FO 957 (Middle East Office).
United States. National Archives and Records Administration
    RG 59 (General Records of the Department of State, 1940–44 and 1945–49).
    RG 84 (Records of the Foreign Service Posts of the Department of State).
    RG 112 (Records of the U.S.A. Typhus Commission).

Private Papers and Diaries

Sir Robin Furness Papers, Private Papers Collection, Middle East Centre, St. Antony's College, Oxford.
Diary of Gertrude Butrus Ghali, privately held by Gertrude Butrus Ghali, Giza, Egypt.
Diary of J. Austin Kerr, Rockefeller Foundation Archives, Tarrytown, N.Y.
Diaries of Lord Killearn (Sir Miles Lampson), 1942–46. Middle East Centre, St. Antony's College, Oxford.
Eric Denholm Pridie Memoir, Durham University, Durham, N.C.
Diary of Fred L. Soper, Rockefeller Foundation Archives, Tarrytown, N.Y.

Government Publications

Egypt, *Annual Report on the Work of the Ministry of Public Health,* Ministry of Public Health, 1942–52.
Egypt, *Madhabit (Parliamentary Records), Chamber of Deputies.*
Egypt, *Madhabit (Parliamentary Records), Senate.*

Egypt, *Taqrir al-jambia* (Report on Gambiae). Ministry of Public Health, 1950.
United Kingdom, Hansard (P. Ford and G. Ford), *Catalogue Breviate of Parliamentary Papers.* Oxford, 1961.
United Kingdom, *House of Commons Parliamentary Papers.*

United Nations Publications

Official Record of the World Health Organization.
World Health Organization Annual Report.
World Health Organization Epidemiological and Vital Statistics Report.
Yearbook of the World Health Organization.

Newspapers and Journals in Arabic Published in Cairo

al-Ahram (The Pyramids)
Akhbar al-Yawm (News of the Day)
Akhir Sa'a (The Latest Hour)
al-Assas (The Foundation)
al-Balagh (The Communiqué)
al-Dustur (The Constitution)
Ikhwan al-Muslimin (daily)
Ikhwan al-Muslimin (weekly)
Ithnayn wa Dunya (Tuesday and the World)
al-Jamahir (The Masses)
al-Kutla (The Bloc)
Misr al-Fattat (Young Egypt)
al-Misri (The Egyptian)
al-Musawwar (The Illustrated)
al-Nadhir
Ruz al-Yusuf (Rose of Joseph)
al-Siyasa (The Politics)
al-Wafd al-Misri (The Egyptian Wafd)

Newspapers and Journals in European Languages

La Bourse égyptienne, Cairo.
Egyptian Gazette, Cairo.
Egyptian Mail, Cairo.
Journal d'Égypte, Cairo.
The Lancet, London.
London Times, London.
Los Angeles Times, Los Angeles.
New York Times, New York.
Progrès égyptien, Cairo.

Dissertations

Badran, Margot. "Huda Sha'rawi and the Liberation of the Egyptian Woman." Ph.D. diss., Oxford Univ., 1977.

Botman, Selma. "Oppositional Politics in Egypt: The Communist Movement, 1936–1954," Ph.D. diss., Harvard Univ., 1984.

Franco-Agudelo, Saul. "El Paludismo en America Latina." Ph.D. diss., Univ. of Xochimilco, 1981.

Mazen, A. K. "Development of the Medical Care Program of the Egyptian Region of the United Arab Republic." Ph.D. diss., Stanford Univ., 1961.

Sonbol, Amira El Azhary. "The Creation of a Medical Profession in Egypt during the Nineteenth Century: A Study in Modernization," Ph.D. diss., Georgetown Univ., 1981.

Tignor, Robert L. "Public Health Administration in Egypt under British Rule, 1882–1914," Ph.D. diss., Yale Univ., 1960.

Interviews, 1982–86

Ihsan Abd al-Qadus, journalist and writer, Cairo.

Abla Sa'id Ahmad, nursing supervisor, Mabarra Hospital, Cairo.

Mustafa Amin, editor in chief, *Akhbar,* Cairo.

Salah Atiyya, consultant, World Health Organization, Alexandria.

Tariq al-Bishri, undersecretary, council of state, Cairo.

Muhyi al-Din Farid, former chief, malaria eradication unit, World Health Organization, currently malaria consultant to health secretariat of the Gulf Arab states, Geneva.

Amin al-Gamal, undersecretary, Ministry of Health, Cairo.

Gertrude Butrus Ghali, member, Red Crescent, Giza.

Muhammad Hasanayn Haykal, journalist and writer, Cairo.

Harry Hoogstraal, entomologist, Naval Medical Research Unit 3, Abbasiyya.

J. Austin Kerr, former Rockefeller Foundation malariologist, Bethesda, Md.

Salih Mar'i, physician and director, Luxor Hospital, Luxor.

Wadud Fayzi Musa, former member, Mabarra Muhammad Ali, Cairo.

Abd al-Azim Ramadan, historian of modern Egypt, Cairo.

Louis A. Riehl, former Rockefeller Foundation entomologist and professor emeritus of entomology, University of California, Riverside, Calif.

Abd al-Aziz Salah, consultant, Naval Medical Research Unit 3, Abbasiyya.

Adil Sabit, journalist, Garden City, Cairo.

Fuad Sirag al-Din, Wafd party leader, Garden City, Cairo.

Hasan Yusuf, former deputy chief of the Egyptian royal cabinet and palace press secretary, Cairo.

Books and Articles in Arabic

Abduh, Sa'id. "Waba' al-kulira al-hali: kayf nasha' wa kayf intishar" (The Current Cholera Epidemic: How It Originated and How It Spread). *Journal of the Royal Egyptian Medical Association* 3, no. 11 (Nov. 1947): 480–99.

al-Bishri, Tariq. *al-Harakat al-siyasiyya fi misr, 1945–1952* (The Political Movement in Egypt, 1945–1952). 2d ed. Beirut: Dar al-Shuruq, 1983.

————. "Misr wa al-thawra al-ijtima'iyya, 1947–1948" (Egypt and the Social Revolution, 1947–1948). *al-Katib* 82 (Jan. 1968): 101–19.

Halim, Asma. *Sitta Ayam fi Sa'id.* Cairo: The New Dawn Publishing House, 1944.

Husayn, Taha. *al-Mu'adhdhabun fi al-'ardh* (The Wretched of the Earth). Cairo: al-Kitab al-fiddiy, 1958.

Mabarrat al-mar'at al-jadida (The New Woman), brochure. Cairo, n.p., n.d.

Murad, Mahmud. *Mustafa Amin wa al-siyasa al-misriyya.* Beirut: al-Maktabat al-'asriyya, 1976.

al-Raf'i, Abd al-Rahman. *Fi aqab al-thawrat al-misriyya* (The Consequences of the Egyptian Revolution), vol. 3. Cairo: Maktabat al-nahda al-misriyya, 1951.

Ramadan, Abd al-Azim. *Tatawwur al-harakat al-wataniyya fi misr, min sanata 1937 ila sanata 1948* (The Development of the National Movement in Egypt from 1937 to 1948). Beirut: al-Watan al-'arabi, 1968.

Yusuf, Hasan. *al-Qasr wa duruhu fi al-siyasat al-misriyya, 1922–1952* (The Palace and Its Role in Egyptian Politics, 1922–1952). Cairo: Markaz al-dirasat al-siyasiya wa al-istratijiya, 1982.

Books and Articles in European Languages

Afifi, A. A., and L. A. Sagan. "Energy and Literacy: An Index of Health Development," unpublished paper. Vienna: International Institute for Applied Systems Analysis, Aug. 1978.

Alport, A. Cecil. *One Hour of Justice: The Black Book of the Egyptian Hospitals and a Fellaheen Charter.* London: Dorothy Crisp and Co. Ltd., 1946.

Ammar, Hamed. *Growing Up in an Egyptian Village: Silwa, Province of Aswan.* London: Routledge & Kegan, 1954.

Arafa, Bahiga. *The Social Activities of the Egyptian Feminist Union.* Cairo: Elias' Modern Press, 1973.

Aronson, Geoffrey. *From Sideshow to Center Stage: U.S. Policy toward Egypt, 1946–1956.* Boulder: Lynne Rienner Publishers, Inc., 1986.

"Award of the Shusha Prize." *Journal of the Egyptian Public Health Association* 43, no. 5 (1968): 418–26.

Ayrout, Henry Habib. *The Egyptian Peasant.* Boston: Beacon Press, 1963.

Baer, Gabriel. *A History of Land Ownership in Modern Egypt, 1800–1950.* London: Oxford Univ. Press, 1962.

Baker, Raymond. *Egypt's Uncertain Revolution under Nasser and Sadat.* Cambridge, Mass.: Harvard Univ. Press, 1978.

al-Barawi, Rashid (Rashed el-Barawy). *The Military Coup in Egypt: An Analytical Study.* Cairo: Renaissance Book Store, 1952.

Beinin, Joel, and Zachary Lockman. *Workers on the Nile: Nationalism, Com-

munism, Islam, and the Egyptian Working Class, 1882–1954. Princeton: Princeton Univ. Press, 1987.

Berkov, Robert. *The World Health Organization: A Study in Decentralized International Administration*. Geneva: Droz, 1957.

Berkow, Robert. *The Merck Manual of Diagnosis and Therapy*, 15th ed. Rahway, N.J.: Merck Sharp & Dohme Research Laboratories, 1987.

Berman, Edward H. *The Influence of the Carnegie, Ford, and Rockefeller Foundations on American Foreign Policy: The Ideology of Philanthropy*. Albany: State Univ. of New York Press, 1983.

Berque, Jacques. *Egypt: Imperialism and Revolution*. Trans. Jean Stewart. London: Faber, 1972.

Biraud, Yves, and P. M. Kaul. *World Health Organization Epidemiological and Vital Statistics Report*. Dec. 1947, 140–52.

Blackman, Winifred. *The Fellahin of Upper Egypt*. London: Harrap, 1927.

Botman, Selma. *The Rise of Egyptian Communism, 1939–1970*. Syracuse: Syracuse Univ. Press, 1988.

Brown, E. Richard. *Rockefeller Medicine Men: Medicine and Capitalism in America*. Berkeley: Univ. of California Press, 1979.

Buechel (Buchel), K. H., ed. *The Chemistry of Pesticides*. New York: Wiley, 1983.

Chedid, Andree. *The Sixth Day*. London: A. Blond, 1962.

Cleaver, Harry. "Malaria, the Politics of Public Health and the International Crisis." *The Review of Radical Political Economics* 9, no. 1 (Spring 1977): 81–103.

Cleland, W. W. *The Population Problem of Egypt*. Lancaster, Pa.: Science Press Co., 1936.

Colombe, Marcel. *L'Évolution de l'Égypte, 1924–1940*. Paris: G. P. Maison-neuve, 1951.

Corner, George W. *A History of the Rockefeller Institute, 1901–1953*. New York: Rockefeller Institute Press, 1964.

Cromer, Lord (Evelyn Baring). *Modern Egypt*. London: Macmillan and Co., 1908.

Daniel, Robert L. *American Philanthropy in the Near East, 1820–1960*. Athens, Ohio: Ohio Univ. Press, 1970.

Davis, Eric. *Challenging Colonialism: Bank Misr and Egyptian Industrialization, 1920–1941*. Princeton: Princeton Univ. Press, 1983.

Deeb, Marius. *Party Politics in Egypt: The Wafd and Its Rivals, 1936–1939*. London: Ithaca Press, 1979.

DeButts, Patricia H. "Egyptian-American Rural Improvement Service: A Point Four Project in Egypt, 1953–1963," unpublished paper. Washington, D.C.: U.S. Agency for International Development, Jan. 1981.

Dekmajian, Hrair. "An Analytical History and Evaluation of the Egyptian-American Rural Improvement Service (EARIS), 1953–1965," unpublished paper. Washington, D.C.: U.S. Agency for International Development, April 1981.

DeNovo, John A. *American Interests in the Middle East, 1900–1939.* Minneapolis: Univ. of Minnesota Press, 1964.

———. "The Culbertson Economic Mission and Anglo-American Tensions in the Middle East, 1944–1945." *Journal of American History* 63 (Dec.–Mar. 1976–77): 913–36.

Deutsch, Albert. "Historical Inter-relationships between Medicine and Social Welfare." *Bulletin of the History of Medicine* 9, no. 5 (May 1942): 485–502.

Doyal, Lesley, with Imogen Pennell. *The Political Economy of Health.* Boston: South End Press, 1979.

Estes, J. Worth, and LaVerne Kuhnke. "French Observations of Disease and Drug Use in Late Eighteenth-Century Cairo." *Journal of the History of Medicine and Allied Sciences* 39, no. 2 (Apr. 1984): 121–52.

Evans, Trefor E., ed. *The Killearn Diaries, 1934–1946: The Diplomatic and Personal Record of Lord Killearn.* London: Sidgwick and Jackson, 1972.

Farid, Muhyi al-Din (Mohyeedin Ahmad Farid). "A Preliminary Note on an Unusual Breeding Place of *Anopheles gambiae* in Egypt," *Journal of the Egyptian Medical Association* 26, no. 4 (Apr. 1943): 126–27.

Fernea, Robert. *Nubians in Egypt: Peaceful People.* Austin: Univ. of Texas Press, 1973.

Fosdick, Raymond B. *The Story of the Rockefeller Foundation.* London: Odhams, 1952.

Franco-Agudelo, Saul. "The Rockefeller Foundation's Antimalarial Program in Latin America: Donating or Dominating?" *International Journal of Health Services* 13, no. 1 (1983): 51–67.

Gallagher, Nancy E. *Medicine and Power in Tunisia, 1780–1900.* Cambridge: Cambridge Univ. Press, 1983.

Garrison, Jean. "Public Assistance in Egypt: An Ideological Analysis." *Middle East Journal* (1978): 279–90.

Gaud, M., Muhammad Khalil (Abd al-Khaliq), and M. Vaucel. "The Evolution of the Epidemic of Relapsing Fever, 1942–1946." *Bulletin of the World Health Organization* 1, no. 2 (1948): 93–101.

Ghali, Mirit Butrus (Mirrit Boutros Ghali). *The Policy of Tomorrow (Siyasat al-Ghad* [Cairo, 1938]). Trans. Ismail R. Faruqi. Washington, D.C.: American Council of Learned Societies, 1953.

———. *Un Programme de reforme agraire pour l'Égypte.* Cairo: Imprimerie Nationale, 1947.

Goodman, Neville. *International Health Organizations and Their Work.* London: J. & A. Churchill, 1951.

Gordon, Joel. "The False Hopes of 1950: The Wafd's Last Hurrah and the Demise of Egypt's Old Order." *International Journal of Middle East Studies* 21, no. 2 (May 1989): 193–214.

Grafftey-Smith, Laurence. *Bright Levant.* London: John Murray, 1970.

Green, Stephen. *International Disaster Relief: Toward a Responsive System.* New York: New York Univ. Press, 1979.

Halawani, A., and A. A. Shawarby. "Malaria in Egypt (History, Epidemiology,

Control and Treatment)." *Egyptian Medical Association Journal* 40, no. 11 (1957): 753–92.

Harrison, Gordon. *Mosquitoes, Malaria, and Man: A History of the Hostilities since 1880.* New York: Dutton, 1978.

Haykal, Muhammad Hasanayn (Mohamed Heikal). *The Cairo Documents: The Inside Story of Nasser and His Relationship with World Leaders, Rebels, and Statesmen.* New York: Doubleday, 1973.

"Health in Egypt: Recommendations for U.S. Assistance." Washington, D.C.: Institute of Medicine, Jan. 1979.

"History of Cholera in Egypt." *British Medical Journal* 1, no. 1 (1951): 688.

Hudson, Michael. *Arab Politics: The Search for Legitimacy.* New Haven, Conn.: Yale Univ. Press, 1977.

Hussein, Ahmed. *Rural Social Welfare Centres in Egypt.* Cairo: Ministry of Social Affairs, 1951.

———. *Social Welfare in Egypt.* Cairo: Ministry of Social Affairs, 1950.

Hussein, Mahmoud. *Class Conflict in Egypt, 1945–1970.* New York: Monthly Review Press, 1977.

Ismael, Tareq Y. *The Middle East in World Politics: A Study in Contemporary International Relations.* Syracuse: Syracuse Univ. Press, 1974.

Issawi, Charles. *Egypt: An Economic and Social Analysis.* London: Oxford Univ. Press, 1947.

———. *Egypt at Mid-Century: An Economic Analysis.* London: Oxford Univ. Press, 1954.

———. *Egypt in Revolution: An Economic Analysis.* London: Oxford Univ. Press, 1963.

Istiphan, Isis. *Directory of Social Agencies in Cairo.* Cairo: American Univ. at Cairo, 1956.

Jagailloux, Serge. "Médecines et santé dans l'Égypte du XIXᵉ siècle." Doc. d'état: Univ. of Paris IV, Sorbonne, 1983.

Jankowski, James P. *Egypt's Young Rebels: "Young Egypt." 1933–1952.* Stanford, Calif.: Hoover Institution, 1975.

Kamal, A. M. (Ahmed Mohamed Kamal). *Epidemiology of Communicable Diseases.* Cairo: Anglo-American Bookshop, 1958.

Kaminer, Wendy. *Women Volunteering: The Pleasure, Pain, and Politics of Unpaid Work from 1830 to the Present.* Garden City, N.Y.: Anchor Press, 1984.

Kerr, J. Austin, ed. *Building the Health Bridge: Selections from the Works of Fred L. Soper.* Bloomington: Indiana Univ. Press, 1970.

Khalid, Khalid Muhammed. *From Here We Start.* Washington, D.C.: American Council of Learned Societies, 1953.

Khalil Abd al-Khaliq (M. Khalil). "The Cholera Epidemic in Egypt in 1947 (A Summary)." *Journal of the Egyptian Medical Association* 31 (Jan. 1948): 15–21.

———. "The Defence of Egypt against Cholera in the Past, Present, and Future." *Journal of the Egyptian Medical Association* 30 (Dec. 1947): 608–55.

———. "The Effect of the Absolute Humidity of the Atmosphere on the First

Wave of the Cholera Epidemic in Egypt in 1947." *Journal of the Egyptian Medical Association* 31 (Jan. 1948): 39–72.

———. "The 1936 Treaty and the Effect of the Second World War on the Health of the Egyptian Nation." *The Journal of the Royal Egyptian Medical Association* 31, no. 1 (Jan. 1948): 1–11.

Kirk, George. *The Middle East in the War*. London and New York: Oxford Univ. Press, 1952.

———. *The Middle East, 1945–1950*. London and New York: Oxford Univ. Press, 1954.

Kraft, Scott. "Malaria: An Old Enemy Rises Again." *Los Angeles Times*, 22 Nov. 1986.

Kuhnke, LaVerne. *Lives at Risk: Public Health in Nineteenth-Century Egypt*. Berkeley: Univ. of California Press, 1989.

Kurdi, A. H. (A. H. Kordi). "Some Observations on the Effect of Cholera Vaccine during the Recent Cholera Epidemic in Egypt." *Journal of the Royal Egyptian Medical Association* 21, no. 2 (Apr. 1948): 289–99.

Lacouture, Jean, and Simonne Lacouture. *Egypt in Transition*. New York: Criterion, 1958.

Landau, Jacob. *Parliaments and Parties in Egypt*. New York: Praeger, 1954.

Laqueur, Walter Z. *Communism and Nationalism in the Middle East*. London: Praeger, 1961.

Lefort, René. *Ethiopia: An Heretical Revolution?* London: Zed Press, 1983.

Lewis, D. J. "A Northern Record of *Anopheles gambiae*." *Royal Entomological Society of London Proceedings*. Ser. B, 11 (1942): 141–42.

Little, Tom. *Modern Egypt*. New York: Ernest Benn, 1967.

Louis, W. Roger. *The British Empire in the Middle East, 1945–1951: Arab Nationalism, the United States, and Postwar Imperialism*. New York: Oxford Univ. Press, 1984.

———. *Imperialism at Bay: The United States and the Decolonization of the British Empire, 1941–1945*. New York: Oxford Univ. Press, 1978.

Mahfouz, Afaf el-Kosheri. *Socialisme et Pouvoir en Égypte*. Paris: R. Pichon and R. Durand-Auzias, 1972.

Mahfouz, Naguib. *The History of Medical Education in Egypt*. Cairo: Government Press at Bulaq, 1935.

———. *The Life of an Egyptian Doctor*. Edinburgh and London: E. & S. Livingston, Ltd., 1956.

Marlow, John. *Anglo-Egyptian Relations, 1800–1953*. London: Cresset Press, 1954.

Marsot, Afaf Lutfi al-Sayyid. *Egypt's Liberal Experiment: 1922–1936*. Berkeley: Univ. of California Press, 1977.

———. *Egypt in the Reign of Muhammad Ali*. Cambridge: Cambridge Univ. Press, 1984.

———. "Egypt's Revolutionary Gentlewomen." In *Women in the Muslim World*, edited by Lois Beck and Nikki Keddie, 261–76. Cambridge, Mass.: Harvard Univ. Press, 1976.

Mayfield, James B. *Rural Politics in Nasser's Egypt: A Quest for Legitimacy.* Austin: Univ. of Texas Press, 1971.

McBride, Barrie St. Clair. *Farouk of Egypt.* London: Robert Hale, 1967.

McNeill, William. *Plagues and Peoples: A History.* Garden City, N.Y.: Doubleday, 1976.

"Medicine in the Land of Pharoes, Ancient and Modern." *Journal of the Egyptian Medical Association* 11, no. 10 (Dec. 1928): 285–356 T.

El-Mehairy, Theresa. *Medical Doctors: A Study of Role Concept and Job Satisfaction; the Egyptian Case.* Leiden: E. J. Brill, 1984.

Milner, A. *England in Egypt.* London: E. Arnold, 1920.

Ministry of Health, Arab Republic of Egypt. *Egyptian Experience in Primary Health Care.* Cairo, n.d.

Mitchell, Richard P. *The Society of the Muslim Brothers.* London: Oxford Univ. Press, 1969.

Monroe, Elizabeth. *Britain's Moment in the Middle East, 1914–1971.* London: Chatto and Windus, 1981.

Naguib, Mohammed. *Egypt's Destiny.* London: Gollancz, 1955.

Nasser, Gamal Abdul. *Egypt's Liberation: The Philosophy of the Revolution.* Washington, D.C.: Public Affairs Press, 1955.

O'Donnell, Charles Peter. *Bangladesh: Biography of a Muslim Nation.* Boulder, Colo.: Westview, 1984.

Ostrander, Susan A. *Women of the Upper Class.* Philadelphia: Temple Univ. Press, 1984.

Owen, Roger. *Cotton and the Egyptian Economy, 1820–1914.* Oxford: Clarendon, 1969.

Pampana, Emilio. *A Textbook of Malaria Eradication.* London and New York: Oxford Univ. Press, 1969.

Phillips, Thomas. "Feminism and Nationalist Politics in Egypt." In *Women in the Muslim World,* edited by Lois Beck and Nikki Keddie, 277–94. Cambridge, Mass.: Harvard Univ. Press, 1976.

Pillsbury, Barbara. *Traditional Health Care in the Near East.* Washington, D.C.: U.S. Agency for International Development, 1983.

Pollitzer, R. *Cholera.* Geneva: World Health Organization, 1959.

al-Ramli, Ali H. (Ali H. el-Ramli). "Clinical Study of 689 Cases of Cholera Isolated in the Abbassia Fever Hospital." *Journal of the Royal Egyptian Medical Association* 31, no. 4 (Apr. 1948): 322–50.

Rasheed, Baheega Sidky, Taheya Mohammed Asfahani, and Samia Sidky Mourad. *The Egyptian Feminist Union.* Cairo: Anglo-American Bookshop, 1973.

Report—Wellcome Trust, 1937–1956. London: The Wellcome Trust, 1957.

Richards, Alan. *Egypt's Agricultural Development, 1800–1980: Technical and Social Change.* Boulder, Colo.: Westview, 1982.

Richmond, J. C. B. *Egypt, 1798–1952: Her Advance towards a Modern Identity.* London: Methuen, 1977.

Riding, Alan. "Nicaragua: A National Mutiny?" *New York Times Sunday Magazine* (30 July 1978): 39–42.

Rouyer, Pierre-Charles. "Notice sur les médicamens usuels des Égyptiens," in *Description de l'Égypte*," état moderne 10 (Paris: l'Imprimerie Impériale, 1809): 217–32.

Rosen, George. "Disease and Social Criticism: A Contribution to a Theory of Medical History." *Bulletin of the History of Medicine* 10 (June 1941): 5–15.

———. *A History of Public Health.* New York: M. D. Publications, 1958.

Russell, Thomas. *Egyptian Service, 1902–1946.* London: Murray, 1949.

El Saadawi, Nawal. *The Hidden Face of Eve: Women in the Arab World.* London: Zed Press, 1980.

Safran, Nadav. *Egypt in Search of Political Community.* Cambridge, Mass.: Harvard Univ. Press, 1961.

Scholch, Alexander. *Egypt for the Egyptians!: The Socio-political Crisis in Egypt, 1878–1882.* London: Ithaca Press, 1981.

Sha'rawi, Huda (Huda Shaarawi). *Harem Years: The Memoirs of an Egyptian Feminist, 1879–1924,* trans., ed., and intro. Margot Badran. London: Virago Press, 1986.

Shawarby, A. A., A. H. Mahdi, and S. Kotla. "Protective Measures against *Anopheles Gambiae* Invasion to UAR." *Journal of the Egyptian Public Health Association* 42, no. 5 (1967): 194–99.

Shawcross, William. *The Quality of Mercy: Cambodia, Holocaust, and Modern Conscience.* New York: Simon and Schuster, 1984.

Shepherd, Jack. *The Politics of Starvation.* New York: Carnegie Endowment for International Peace, 1975.

Shidrawi, G. R. "Report on a Mission to Upper Egypt and Sudan in Connection with *A. Gambiae* (Arabiensis) Protective and Control Measures," unpublished paper. Cairo: World Health Organization, July 1980.

Shusha, Ali Tawfiq (Aly Tewfik Shousha). "Species-Eradication: The Eradication of *Anopheles gambiae* from Upper Egypt, 1942–1945." *Bulletin of the World Health Organization* 1, no. 2 (1948): 309–52.

———. "Cholera Epidemic in Egypt (1947): A Preliminary Report." *Bulletin of the World Health Organization* 1, no. 2 (Nov. 1948): 353–81.

Siba'i, D. M. (D. M. Sebai). "History of the Evolution of the Department of Public Health in Egypt." *Journal of the Egyptian Medical Association* 11, no. 10 (Dec. 1928): 357–67.

Stephens, Lynn H., and Stephen J. Green. *Disaster Assistance: Appraisal, Reform and New Approaches.* New York: New York Univ. Press, 1979.

Terry, Janice J. *Cornerstone of Egyptian Political Power: The Wafd, 1919–1952.* London: Third World Center, 1979.

Tignor, Robert L. *Modernization and British Colonial Rule in Egypt, 1882–1914.* Princeton: Princeton Univ. Press, 1966.

———. *State, Private Enterprise, and Economic Change in Egypt, 1918–1952.* Princeton: Princeton Univ. Press, 1984.

Umar, Muhammad al-Sayyid (Omar, Mohammed El-Sayed). "Cholera." Handwritten manuscript. Cairo, n.d.

United States Information Bulletin. Cairo, September 1947.

van Heyningen, W. E., and John R. Seal. *Cholera: The American Scientific Experience, 1947–1980.* Boulder, Colo.: Westview, 1983.

Vatikiotis, P. J. *The Modern History of Egypt.* Baltimore: Johns Hopkins Univ. Press, 1985.

Walker, John. *Folk Medicine in Modern Egypt.* London: Luzac, 1934.

Warburg, Gabriel R. *Egypt and the Sudan: Studies in History and Politics.* London: Cass, 1985.

Weir, J. M. "An Evaluation of Health and Sanitation in Egyptian Villages." *Journal of the Egyptian Public Health Association* 27, no. 3 (1952): 55–119.

Wilmington, Martin W. *The Middle East Supply Centre.* Albany: State Univ. of New York Press, 1971.

World Health Organization. *The First Ten Years of the World Health Organization.* Geneva, 1958.

Worthington, E. B. *Middle East Science: A Survey of Subjects Other than Agriculture.* London: H. M. Stationery Office, 1946.

Zaghloul, Ahmed Zaher (Ahmad Zahir Zaghloul). "Rural Health Services in U.A.R." *Journal of the Egyptian Public Health Association* 38, no. 5 (1963): 217–42.

Zayid, Mahmud Y. *Egypt's Struggle for Independence.* Beirut: Khayats, 1965.

Films

Shahin, Yusuf (Youssef Chahine). *Yawm al-sadis* (The Sixth Day). Cairo, 1986.

Salah, Tawfiq. *Sira' al-Abtal* (Struggle of Heroes). Cairo, 1962.

Index

Abaza, Fikri, 161

Abbasiyya, 27

Abbasiyya Fever Hospital: American presence at, 104, 128, 165; cholera studies at, 138, 165; malaria at, 190n.83; new buildings at, 103; volunteers at, 135

Abbud, Ahmad, 45

Abbud, Jemima, 45, 61, 91, 93

Abbud Pasha, 81

Abd al-Hadi, Ibrahim, 88, 93, 103, 161, 168

Abd al-Khaliq, Khalil: anti-British attitude of, 99, 114, 151–56; and malaria, 34, 73; quarantine duties of, 21, 93; and Soper, 28

Abd al-Qadus, Ihsan, 49–50

Abdin Palace, 90

Abduh, Sa'id, 121, 154, 155

Adisat, 71, 81

Afifi, M. M., 50

Africa, 102, 150, 174; central, 93; East, 84; North, 114; sub-Saharan, 5, 14, 86; West, 23, 24, 28

Agrarian Reform, 69

Agriculture, 13–14, 33, 56, 172, 174. *See also* Irrigation

Ahmad, Abla Sa'id, 41, 43, 171

Ahmad, Samira, 174

al-Ahram: coverage of cholera, 130, 141, 154; coverage of malaria, 26, 38, 48, 62, 63, 73

Aisha, Princess, 93

Akhbar al-Yawm: coverage of cholera, 141, 142, 143, 150; coverage of sanitation, 120; criticism of Zionism, 130

Akhir Sa'a: coverage of cholera, 119, 134; coverage of malaria, 48, 52; coverage of public health, 161; coverage of sanitation, 120

Allah, Hasan Khayr, 141

Allah, Ragab Hasan Khayr, 141

Alexandria, 124, 126, 128, 132

Allied troops: danger of malaria to, 23, 26, 29, 77; occupation of Egypt by, 21, 27, 29, 99

American Red Cross, 47, 85

American University, 15

Amin, Mustafa, 41, 47, 54, 59, 64–65

Amin, Ni'matullah, 41, 48

Ammar, Hamed, 37

Ancylostomiasis, 12, 15. *See also* Hookworm

Anglo-Egyptian Union, 91

Anopheles gambiae, 4, 14, 57, 70, 80, 89; breeding of, 21–25, 36, 73, 81; eradication of, 28–29, 32, 35–39, 81–82, 86, 92–94, 117–78, 188n.26; source of, 73, 93, 150. *See also* Mosquitoes

Anopheles pharoensis, 4, 14, 21

Anopheles sergenti, 4

Antibiotics, 138

Arab League, 130

Armant, 45, 81, 89, 92

Asad, Fakhri, 125

Ashur, Badrawi, 134–35

Asia, 5, 114, 174

Asiut: Mabarra Muhammad Ali in, 108, 111; mosquito discovered in, 21; Nahhas visit to, 71; Rockefeller Foundation headquarters in, 86, 89, 90, 93

al-Assas, 131, 155

Aswan dam: completion of, 6, 172; electrification by, 66; raising of, 23, 26, 61

Aswan province, 24, 58; economic conditions in, 46, 51, 65–67; malaria in, 21, 31–32, 61, 89, 126, 148; relief in, 31–32, 37, 52, 71–73, 81, 94

al-Aswani, Abbas, 125

Atabrine: discovery of, 187n.16; distribution of, 32, 34, 36, 61, 88, 90, 190n.69; supply of, 60, 61, 88, 90

Atiyya, Salah, 155

Avierino, Mr., 135

Ayn Shams University, 156

Ayrout, Habib, 120, 160

Egypt's Other Wars was composed in 10 on 13.5 Galliard on a Mergenthaler Linotron 202 by Brevis Press; printed by sheet-fed offset on 60-pound, acid-free Glatfelter Natural, and Smyth-sewn and bound over binder's boards in Holliston Roxite, by Braun-Brumfield, Inc.; with dust jackets printed in 1 color by Braun-Brumfield, Inc.; designed by Kachergis Book Design of Pittsboro, North Carolina; and published by Syracuse University Press, Syracuse, New York 13244-5160